Analysis of Waiting-Time Data in Health Services Research

Boris Sobolev · Lisa Kuramoto

Analysis of Waiting-Time Data in Health Services Research

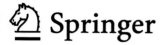 Springer

Boris Sobolev
University of British Columbia
Department of Health Care and Epidemiology
5804 Fairview Avenue
Vancouver, BC V6T 1Z3
Canada
sobolev@interchange.ubc.ca

Lisa Kuramoto
Vancouver Coastal Health Research Institute
Centre for Clinical Epidemiology & Evaluation
828 West 10th Avenue
Vancouver, BC V5Z 1L8
Canada
lisa.kuramoto@vch.ca

ISBN: 978-0-387-76421-4   e-ISBN: 978-0-387-76422-1

Library of Congress Control Number: 2007940842

Printed on acid-free paper.

9 8 7 6 5 4 3 2 1

springer.com

To Peter Brown, a vascular surgeon

Preface

In health care systems that provide universal access to care, efforts to contain costs for standby hospital capacity usually result in wait lists for surgical procedures. When access to health care is rationed by such wait lists, the length of time that patients are required to wait is usually uncertain. This uncertainty is a natural product of stochastic variation in service time and in the percentage of urgent cases in any queuing system. However, in a queue for elective (nonemergency) procedures, waiting-time uncertainty has many additional causes. For instance, decisions of both patients and care providers may override a queue discipline. Alternatively, the lack of a hospital resource, such as beds in the intensive care unit, may change queuing practices in favor of services that would not require the resource.

Waiting time is often compared between regions, hospitals, periods, or surgical services to evaluate policy and performance. However, surprisingly little attention has been given to the variation in times spent in a single queue. Why some patients wait longer than others remains an important question in health services research. It is unclear, for example, whether time to service varies more than would be expected through chance alone after differences in clinical condition are taken into account. Another important issue is preferential allocation of hospital resources. It also remains unclear whether patients of low priority are admitted directly as a way to circumvent long wait lists or to substitute for cancellations on the operating room schedule. Wait lists for elective surgery have typically been accepted on the premise that they ensure the most efficient use of hospital resources; the only alternative would be underutilization of capacity within the health care system. Recently, however, the debate has shifted toward the issue of how much capacity is required to maintain safe wait lists. Policy makers have called for establishing target access times for major operations that would minimize the adverse events associated with treatment delay.

Although it was recognized early that methods of time-to-event analysis are applicable to waiting-time data, literature on the methodology of collecting, reporting, and analyzing waiting times is scarce, in particular for applications of competing-risks methods. The purpose of this book is to place the analysis of waiting-time data within the paradigm of health services research, the study of outcomes of health care delivery to a population. We suggest two uses for this book. First, it is intended as a reference for health services researchers who are looking for statistical tools with which to study waiting times for health services. The book provides coverage of statistical concepts and methods for the analysis and interpretation of waiting-time data, such as time-to-event analysis, discrete-time regression models, competing risks, and pseudovalues regression models. Second, the book is a workbook for a range of professionals in the health-care community, offering a collection of examples of waiting-time data analysis in health services research. It gives a practical perspective, from framing the study question through interpretation of results, on how to describe and compare waiting experiences, how to study the impact of factors associated with waiting times, and how to use appropriate statistical techniques.

The book is divided into 10 chapters, grouped in two parts. Part I, Data, Questions and Methods, introduces the field of health services research on access to care. Chapter 1 provides a comprehensive overview of waiting-time data in health services research. In particular, we describe types of data and types of questions, study designs, and options for analysis of waiting-time data. We then develop the statistical rationale for evaluating the effects of factors potentially associated with waiting times in surgical care by defining a study outcome admission from the wait list. Arguing that scheduling the operation provides a single opportunity for admission, we develop a measure of access to elective procedures the probability of admission per scheduling cycle. We observe that because factors interfering with access may lower chances of admission, it is possible to study their impact on access to service by estimating the probability of admission across categories of explanatory variables. The effects of study variables can be further estimated by modeling the probability of admission as a function of study variables. In Chapter 2, we described three sets of records on access to surgery at the hospital, regional, and population level, respectively, which are used for the analyses in Part II. Chapter 3 presents statistical methods for the analysis of waiting-time data. We first introduce the descriptive statistics that are used to summarize the frequency of events on wait lists, such as proportions, event rates, and cumulative incidence functions. In particular, we show that measuring the proportion of patients admitted within certain time frames may shed light on how factors within and outside elective care influence the probability of access to service. We then discuss measures of comparison and introduce corresponding tests for comparing these measures statistically across groups. Finally, we describe regression models that are used to quantify the effects of explanatory variables on wait-list outcomes. For each model we show how to interpret the regression coefficients.

Part II, Waiting-time Studies, presents case studies of waiting-time data, in which we address the questions posed in Part I. In particular, in Chapter 3 we show the use of waiting-time data to estimate admission probabilities and to study variation in waiting times within a single queue. In the chapters that follow, we show statistical techniques appropriate for gaining a better understanding of the relation between weekly number of emergency referrals and rate of elective admissions within the target access time, the proportion of patients who undergo late surgery after registration on surgical wait lists of different sizes, the effect of delays in scheduling an operation on waiting time for surgery, and the risk of unplanned emergency surgery among patients waiting for elective surgery, among other issues.

The data analyses and output presented in this book were generated using SAS/STAT software from the SAS System for Windows, version 9.1.3. Matlab version 7.0.1 from MathWorks, Inc. was used to generate the figures presented in this book and perform some statistical analyses. The appendix contains the SAS codes and macros that we developed for preparing the data sets described in Part I, as well as the SAS and Matlab codes for performing some of the statistical analyses in Part II.

The writing of this book was made possible, in part, through funding from the Canada Research Chairs Program. We gratefully acknowledge the support of the Centre for Clinical Epidemiology & Evaluation at the Vancouver Coastal Health Research Institute, where most of the research was undertaken, and the able assistance of Peggy Robinson and Taina Immonen in preparing the manuscript.

Innovations in health care management require leadership. We dedicate this book to Dr. Peter Brown, a valued leader who championed the Change Foundation Waiting List Project that gave birth to wait-list management systems in the network of regional hospitals in Ontario, Canada.

Vancouver, British Columbia   *Boris Sobolev*
September 2007   *Lisa Kuramoto*

Contents

Part I Data, Questions and Methods

Part II Waiting-time Studies

List of Tables

List of Figures

Data, Questions and Methods

1

Health services research on access to care

1.1 Access to elective care

In this book, we focus on access to elective surgical procedures provided in hospital operating rooms. Access to patient care at hospitals is usually managed by scheduling demands for service. In the scheduling of surgical demand, the patients available for the next service period are identified, and hospital resources are reserved to ensure appropriate care before and after an instance of surgery [16]. To plan utilization of surgical suite resources, the hospital releases, on a periodic basis, blocks of operating room time to various surgical services, each of which then places its patients on the operating room schedule [77]. Some time slots are set aside for emergency cases. Any time not booked by a service is made available to other services. We use the term *scheduling cycle* for the sequence of events in surgical scheduling between two consecutive releases of operating time blocks.

Within services, patients are selected from wait lists and scheduled for surgery on the basis of urgency, best use of allocated operating time, and availability of hospital resources. However, emergency patients have preferential access to hospital resources, which may lead to cancellation of scheduled operations. Conversely, already scheduled patients may undergo surgery ahead of their scheduled dates if an operating room time slot becomes available, especially if they can come in at very short notice. Service access is defined as *immediate* if patients are admitted within the scheduling cycle that started before they were put on the wait list. Access is said to be *delayed* if patients were admitted within the scheduling cycle that started after their acceptance for service.

1.2 Wait lists

Patients are placed on a wait list after the decision to perform surgery is made, but only if they cannot be immediately added to the current operating room schedule. Patients are ranked by how urgently they need treatment, and a priority group is assigned to each patient to determine relative position on the list. Patients with a higher priority will be selected for service ahead of those with a lower priority, regardless of when they were placed on the list. Patients in the same priority group are ranked in order of arrival time.

Before being added to the operating room schedule, each patient is assessed by his or her surgeon to determine suitability for surgery. If a patient is deemed unfit, scheduling of the operation may be postponed. Scheduling the operation may be delayed for the following additional reasons: the patient decides to postpone the surgery; the hospital ward, bed, or operating room is unavailable at the scheduled time; or the doctor decides to send the patient for additional preoperative investigation.

Patients are removed from the wait list after undergoing the operation; if they die while awaiting surgery, reconsider the decision to undergo surgery, decline admission, accept surgery from another surgeon, or move out of the province; if their condition deteriorates to the point that the operation is no longer possible; if the operation is deferred or suspended on medical grounds; if the physician decides to try a medical treatment instead of waiting for surgery; if their condition precludes scheduling surgery; if their condition improves and surgery becomes unnecessary; or if the operation no longer offers the likelihood of improvement. Patients may eventually be reinstated on the list following medical deferral, self-deferral, or failure to attend [11].

1.3 Waiting times

Waiting, or staying in a queue, refers to the time between entering and leaving the queue. In elective medical services, waiting time generally refers to the interval between acceptance and admission for service. Registration on the wait list is clearly the appropriate event to denote the patient's acceptance to receive service. Other events, such as the decision to perform surgery expressed in a letter to the patient's referring physician, a final visit to a specialist, or facility booking are used as proxies only if the date of registration on the wait list is not available [99].

Although the event of admission ends waiting in a queue, the majority of waiting-time studies have used the date of surgery to denote the end of the waiting period [35]. This option has been chosen either because of study design (where only those patients who underwent the procedure were eligible for a study) or data availability. We believe that admission to hospital characterizes the end of the waiting experience better than the receipt of the surgical service because time from admission to service usually includes several procedures that prepare a patient for the service. In addition, more than one service can take place during the same admission, and even though the services are provided on different days, waiting is essentially over on the date of the admission.

One scheduling cycle serves as the natural counting unit for time to admission because only scheduling generates elective admission; it thus provides a single opportunity for admission to occur. Therefore, in studies on access to elective care, time to admission is inherently discrete and is best measured as the number of new scheduling cycles from registration to admission. If scheduling is done weekly, waiting time may be computed as the number of calendar weeks between registration and admission. For those removed from the wait list before admission, the waiting time is then computed as the number of calendar weeks from registration to removal.

If the goal is to capture the total duration of waiting, the time between registration and admission is computed irrespective of events that take place within that period. The other approach is to "restart the clock" if a patient comes off the list temporarily but is then reinstated; the patient is thus considered to have had more than one waiting episode. Instances when the patient self-defers, or fails to attend should be differentiated from instances when the operation is deferred or suspended on medical grounds.

1.4 Studies of waiting times

The overall purpose of a waiting-time study is to estimate parameters of access to care that can be compared between providers, periods, or management practices. The results of several studies highlight the need for a waiting-time registry to collect prospective data on patient progress in a queue from acceptance for treatment

[118]. Such a registry helps in monitoring critical events during a stay in the queue and would record reasons for leaving the queue. Use of a population-based registry would also facilitate collecting information to account for differences in service demand between population groups. In the absence of a prospective registry, service records allow us to ascertain waiting times for patients who are eventually admitted. However, such records have the potential for selection bias, because those who do not attend, those who self-defer, and those whose surgery is suspended on medical or administrative grounds are not represented [10]. Because the timing of a service in a queue is random, statistical models for service rates are drawn from the general area of time-to-event analysis [53]. The chief analytical tool in such analyses is the access function, that is, the probability of accessing a service within a certain time of registration on the wait list [78], which is a useful way of describing the proportion of those in a queue who were served as a function of wait-list time [11]. Comparing access probabilities by study factors allows measurement of their effects on access to care.

1.5 Factors associated with waiting times

Factors that may affect time to admission can be classified into four groups: demands, hospital resources, waiting-list management, and patient characteristics.

Although the level of demand may be regarded as largely external to the processes by which patients gain access to service from waiting lists, variations in time of arrival among patients undergoing elective surgery and variations in the needs of these patients may create opportunities for speeding up or delaying access. For instance, treatment of emergency cases may cause cancellation of planned elective services, or patients may put demands on hospital resources different from those anticipated. Therefore, a batch arrival or a prolonged series of patients with the same needs may extend waits. Another factor to be considered is the manner in which the arrival pattern changes over time [11].

The simple measure of arrival rates, according to type of surgical demand, is useful in comparative studies. If an arrival pattern changes from one calendar year to the next, period-specific arrival rates should be taken into account. Longitudinal records of resource availability, such as the split of operating room hours between emergency and elective cases, bed vacancies, and the number of anesthesiologists, are instrumental for creating time-dependent covariates. If detailed records of the status of resources are not available, the average numbers during a calendar period might be used.

The availability of hospital resources, such as surgeons, anesthesiologists, surgical nurses, operating rooms, special equipment, and beds, defines the chances of a patient being placed on the surgical schedule [16]. Therefore, it is important to include resource-related indicators in analyzing whether differences in availability of resources, as opposed to differences in management practices, can explain variations in access to care [99].

The most important management-related factor is the priority discipline by which patients are selected for scheduling once a queue has formed. As noted above, patients with a higher priority are usually selected ahead of those with a lower priority, regardless of when they were added to the list, and patients in the same priority group are usually selected in the order of their arrival. However, there are several situations in which this priority discipline may be altered. In the first, which is called preemptive queue, an emergency patient might be allowed to enter the service immediately upon arrival, even if an elective patient has already been admitted to hospital. The second situation is related to the management practice based on the current state of the schedule and the queue. The need to avoid idle operating room time, which may occur if planned elective surgery is cancelled, creates opportunities for the immediate admission of purely elective cases. If operating room time becomes available unexpectedly, surgeons for whom the operating room time was allocated ask managers to find out if anyone on the list can come in at short notice. Therefore, demand on different hospital resources and the availability of those resources may change the queue discipline in favor of less urgent cases or late cases in the same priority group.

The number of priority groups might be an important factor, given that variation in waiting times tends to decline within each group. Usually each priority group has a target access time, but this target time might be a continuous variable if it is directly related to an urgency score calculated by a formal algorithm [61]. Therefore, the range of target access times within each priority group could be important in explaining variability in waiting time. Another important characteristic of queuing procedures is whether patients are partitioned to create a pool for immediate substitution when an operation on the current schedule is cancelled. Patients may be asked in advance if they are able to come in at very short notice, especially if the procedure requires no preparatory work-up. This effectively divides a queue into two pools according to patients' agreement to come in at short notice. Therefore, such a policy may change the first-come, first-served discipline within priority groups.

There are two types of management policy for cancellations of booked services. In the first type, patients are taken off the list and reinstated later. In the second type, patients are kept on the list until their eventual admission, irrespective of events taking place between acceptance and admission. Therefore, comparisons between providers may produce biased results if intermediate events occurring between registration and admission are not taken into account.

Surgical needs, severity of the patient's condition, and the presence of comorbidity are the most important patient-related factors. Comorbidity denotes the presence of one or more diseases in addition to the disease under study. In general, a large number of comorbid conditions is a contraindication to aggressive treatment and may jeopardize the likelihood of treatment success. Other patient-related factors are whether the patient was reinstated on the list after earlier removal because of cancellation, whether the patient was placed on the list from a follow-up program, whether the patient was waiting for a second procedure, and whether the patient was in a short-notice pool. Age and sex are important confounding factors because of their association with surgical need. Differences in access to treatment among social classes could also be relevant to a waiting-time study [88]. It has been suggested that better-educated patients may receive referral to specialist services for less critical conditions, at earlier stages, and with lower levels of expected benefits [98]. In addition, members of groups with higher socioeconomic status may have the skills required to negotiate expedited access to care [79].

Patients may also be treated differently depending on where they live. Therefore, differences in referral patterns (that is, differences between referring physicians as to the stages of disease at which they think it is appropriate to refer patients to hospital) and variations in clinical practice in the assessment of urgency must be considered in waiting-time studies [19]. The nonclinical factors that may operate as confounders include the hospital affiliation of the referring physicians [6] and preferential allocation of hospital resources [5].

1.6 Types of data

Waiting-time studies may be classified as either prospective or retrospective according to how waiting time is ascertained. In a prospective study, where waiting time is evaluated from registration to admission or removal from the list for a reason other than admission, the sampling unit is "patient listed". In a retrospective study, where waiting time is ascertained from admission backward to some preceding moment, the sampling unit is "patient admitted". Whereas prospective studies examine how long patients who have been *accepted* for treatment wait for admission to hospital, retrospective studies examine how long patients who have been *admitted* were required to wait after registration.

1.6.1 Prospective registries

A waiting-time registry facilitates the collection of prospective information on events and circumstances that have led to admission or removal within a cohort of patients recruited to the waiting list [84]. In the absence of waiting-time registries, service or admission records collected in administrative databases are often used to select patients for study [76]. If every wait ended in admission, the two sources would generate equivalent data. However, neither patients removed before admission nor those still waiting are represented in service records [35].

The data sets from a prospective registry offer a valid method of calculating waiting times that ensures complete representation of the experience of patients: those who were accepted over a given period, those awaiting attention at a particular moment, those who underwent treatment during a specified period, and those who were removed from the wait list without treatment.

1.6.2 Operating room records

Registration for a service is the point at which clinicians confirm the need for treatment and service providers begin planning resource allocation for admission. However, at many hospitals, patients are not represented in the operating room records until the treatment has taken place. In time-to-event studies in other fields, it has been suggested that such a retrospective design can lead to serious problems with inferences [121]. Retrospective design can similarly bias the results of a waiting-time study. For instance, the waiting times of patients placed on the list late in the study will necessarily be short. Thus, the effect of factors associated with long waits would be biased toward the null, whereas the effect of urgency status would be overestimated. Even if patient removals occurred at random, discarding those removed from the waiting list before surgery would invalidate the results of a study. For instance, coexisting illnesses may delay surgery in one group but have no effect in another. If sicker patients are routinely removed from a queue before admission, there is a potential for bias in a between-group comparison.

1.6.3 Wait-list counts

Wait-list censuses provide information on how long patients currently on a list have been waiting [38]. This cross-sectional design also involves opportunities for selection bias, and patients with long waits are over-represented [10]. For this book, we used primarily data sets containing records of registrations rather than records of admission for service, although we do compare the service- and registration-based approaches.

1.7 Types of questions

Waiting lists for elective surgery have been commonly accepted in publicly funded health care systems on the premise that they ensure the most efficient use of hospital resources; the only alternative would be underutilization of capacity within the system [81]. The system's operational considerations alone may be irrelevant, in that long waiting times constitute deprivation of rights to personal inviolability. The debate has therefore shifted toward the issue of how much capacity is required to maintain safe wait lists. Many governments have called for target access times for surgical procedures that would minimize the adverse events associated with treatment delay. A major effort has been devoted to understanding why some patients wait longer than others for the same service. In the following sections we introduce some questions that have been considered in studies on access to care.

1.7.1 What is the variation in time spent waiting for elective surgery?

The length of time that patients spend on wait lists has been examined in several studies that have reported on variations in waiting times according to procedure, urgency, practice, period, and type of surgical service. Few studies have been concerned with the variation in waits for services from a single provider, although this information is important for understanding what factors are involved. Most studies are primarily concerned with the statistical variation in a queue of patients with equal surgical needs and urgency. Whether waiting times vary by chance alone after adjustment for clinical factors, variation in demand, and patient and hospital characteristics remains an important question in health services research on access to surgery.

1.7.2 What is the probability of undergoing surgery within a certain time?

In any analysis of hospital wait lists, it is useful to obtain the probability distribution of waiting times so that the proportion of listed patients undergoing treatment within a certain period can be compared between services, calendar years, and management practices. This probability distribution allows researchers to compare performance in terms of the percentage of patients who had a specified wait (for example, 0 to 2 months) in two periods. Alternatively, services can be compared by wait-list times for a specified percentile of waiting times, for example, the 50th percentile.

1.7.3 Does priority affect chances of admission for surgery?

Explicitly queuing patients who are awaiting elective surgery according to urgency of required treatment is generally perceived as a suitable method to facilitate access to care within a clinically appropriate time frame. Most surgical queue-management systems use clinical criteria to determine the urgency of the need for a procedure [86]. In theory, patients are prioritized according to established guidelines, and access to surgery is expedited if they are considered at greater risk of deterioration or death. However, wide variations in individual waiting times have been reported within priority groups [84]. This may suggest that priority ranking serves only as an aid in queuing patients for elective surgery, with the decisions of patients, surgeons, and service managers easily altering the order of admissions. Indeed, patients may be selected for surgery on the basis of best use of allocated operating room time, availability of hospital resources, or anticipated length of stay in intensive care. Therefore, several studies have estimated the probability of undergoing surgery as a function of wait-list time in a synthetic cohort of patients registered on priority wait lists. In Part II we report on the impact of priority, using an example from vascular surgery, where the urgency of intervention can be clearly defined.

1.7.4 Does registration period affect waiting times?

Concerned with growing wait lists for cardiac surgery in the mid-1990s, the provincial government in British Columbia, Canada, started providing supplementary funding to increase the annual number of coronary artery bypass grafting (CABG) procedures by 15%, starting in 1998. Although they were intended to improve the situation, it is not known whether these measures changed the time that patients spent on wait lists for elective CABG.

Previous studies have shown inconsistent results regarding the impact of supplementary funding on time to surgery in publicly funded health care systems [99]. It has been suggested that the effect may vary according to the scope (single hospital versus all hospitals in a region) and the term (one-time versus ongoing increases) of funding commitment [57]. In addition, there has been little information on the impact of supplementary funding across different priority groups.

In Part II, Chapter 6, we describe one study that compared the number of weeks between being registered for CABG and undergoing the operation for equal proportions of patients registered in different years before and after the provincial government started providing supplementary funding [70]. The specific research questions were (1) Did the period of registration affect the time that patients spent on wait lists for CABG? and (2) Was the period effect similar across priority groups?

1.7.5 Does the type of procedure affect waiting times?

Although access to surgery depends on the assigned priority, several studies have reported that patients with equal surgical needs have waited considerably different times for elective procedures provided by a single surgical service [103]. For example, in Canadian hospitals, the department of vascular surgery performs a variety of surgical procedures, such as abdominal aortic aneurysm repair, carotid endarterectomy, peripheral vascular bypass surgery, other arterial reconstructive and graft procedures involving blood supply to the legs, and creation of arteriovenous fistula to provide long-term access for hemodialysis in patients with renal failure. Patients waiting for these procedures compete for the same hospital resources. If operating room time becomes available unexpectedly, surgeons ask the office managers to find out if anyone can come in within a few hours, especially for a procedure requiring no preparatory work-up. On the other hand, cancellations because of lack of a hospital resource, such as an intensive care unit bed, can schedule first procedures that do not require the resource. Therefore, the question is often asked whether the type of procedure has an independent effect on services where queuing procedures are in place [27].

1.7.6 Does wait-list size at registration affect time to surgery?

The length of a surgical wait list is a common surrogate for the expected wait for hospital admission. Indeed, if there are patients already on the list, a patient who has just arrived will be admitted within a certain period only if all current patients have been served during that period. In British Columbia, priority wait lists are commonly used to manage access to elective procedures according to urgency of need for treatment. In particular, patients with coronary artery disease are prioritized according to angina symptoms, coronary anatomy, and impairment of left ventricular function to facilitate access to surgical revascularization within a clinically appropriate time. Describing waiting times for CABG in the province, Katz et al. suggested that variation in the size of the wait list among individual surgeons may be an important factor as well [60]. Surprisingly little is known about how the list size at registration affects waiting time for elective surgical procedures. Without this information, it is difficult to accurately estimate how much service capacity is required to maintain short wait lists for surgery [119].

1.7.7 What is the relation between emergency referrals and elective admission within the target time?

Comparing the proportions of patients who undergo elective surgery within the target access time across hospitals may be misleading if referral patterns are not considered. At least one study found that variations in outpatient referral rates were an important determinant of variations in admission rates [30]. Given its association with variations in practice, referral pattern is a potential confounding factor for any observed associations between practice patterns and performance indicators. Little is known about the relation between volume of emergency referrals and admission rates from a waiting list for the same surgical service, although a batch arrival or a prolonged series of emergency cases would seem likely to delay access for patients already on the list. In theory, queuing procedures may ensure equal access to care according to patient need and urgency, if implemented uniformly across the health care system. However, the chances of admission for elective surgery can easily be altered if surgical services experience an uneven influx of emergency cases [107]. For instance, the availability of hospital resources may require to serve less urgent cases first [16], or emergency cases may lead to cancellation of planned elective services, even though some time slots on the operating room schedule are usually set aside for emergency procedures [77]. For evaluation purposes therefore the common concern is whether the proportions of patients who undergo surgery within the target access time can be accurately estimated without considering emergency caseload.

1.7.8 What proportion of patients have late surgery after registration on wait lists of different sizes?

The proportion of patients who undergo surgery within a clinically acceptable time is an important performance indicator in health care systems that use wait lists to manage access to care [118]. In theory, queuing procedures should ensure access to care according to urgency of treatment if implemented uniformly. Sobolev et al. performed an empirical analysis of a population-based registry and found that the length of the queue at registration affected the time to elective surgery [112]. Surprisingly little is known about how the list size at registration affects the chances of undergoing elective surgical procedures within an acceptable time. The common concern for evaluation purposes is therefore whether the proportion of late surgeries can be accurately estimated without considering the length of the wait list. In Part II, Chapter 7 of this volume, we describe a study that aimed to determine the proportion of patients who had late surgery after registration on surgical wait lists of different sizes.

1.7.9 What is the effect of delays in scheduling an operation?

When time to elective admission is compared between providers, periods, or management practices to evaluate performance, there is a possibility that patients will have experienced an intermediate event between registration and admission for treatment. Such intermediate events might include a delay in scheduling the operation, cancellation of booked services, or reinstatement after self-deferral. The occurrence of the events preceding admission may alter the admission rate in one group, having no effect in the other; may have the same effect in both groups; or may have different effects in each group. The common concern is therefore the potential bias in estimates of relative admission rates when the comparison is done without considering events preceding admission. There is a strong argument that an adjustment should be performed for time-varying covariates when studying differences between groups in a prospective study [62].

In Part II, Chapter 7 of this volume, we assess the magnitude of the bias when access to surgery is compared between two registration periods without data on intermediate events. The aim is to demonstrate the effect of exclusion of data on delays in scheduling operations in calculating differences in admission rates. Waiting-time analysis was conducted in two ways: first, with data on elective admission only and then with additional data on the occurrence and timing of delay in scheduling the operation.

1.7.10 Do longer delays contribute to preoperative mortality among patients with less urgent need for surgery?

In surgical care, the existence of wait lists for elective procedures raise concerns about delaying necessary treatment. Explicitly queuing patients with coronary artery disease according to urgency is generally perceived as a method of facilitating access to treatment within a clinically appropriate time. As such, priority wait lists manage delays by prioritizing patients by need. For example, when accepting patients on CABG wait lists in British Columbia, cardiac surgeons indicate the priority for booking the operating room according to angina symptoms, coronary anatomy, and left ventricular function.

Although several studies have described the impact of prioritization on time to surgery [33, 101], the effects of sharing services between patients with different priorities are less well understood. In particular, little attention has been given to the impact of delaying low-risk patients to expedite treatment of those at higher risk.

In a patient with coronary artery disease who is to undergo CABG, delaying that operation may lead to deterioration of the patient's condition, a poor clinical outcome, and an increased risk of death. In population-based studies, death before CABG has been reported in 0.4% to 1.3% of patients in whom it was felt that surgery could be safely delayed. These estimates, however, are affected by the incidence of both surgery and death. Therefore, without further analysis seeking to isolate the effect of these two competing risks, it is not clear whether longer delays contribute to the probability of death before surgery among patients in the less urgent category.

From a methodological perspective, measuring mortality on surgical wait lists is similar to quantifying risk of death over time in populations exposed to competing risks [1]. The time-dependent cumulative incidence of preoperative death, which accounts for the occurrence and timing of competing events, is a useful way of comparing the proportion of patients who die before surgery across urgency groups [45].

1.7.11 What is the risk of unplanned emergency surgery among patients waiting for surgery?

In patients with coronary artery disease for whom elective surgical revascularization is indicated, extended treatment delays may increase the probability of emergency admission [94]. Unplanned admission may be associated with an episode of unstable angina or aggravation of symptoms requiring immediate admission to hospital [68]. The proportion of patients who undergo elective surgery through unplanned emergency admission was identified as an important performance indicator in health care systems that use wait lists to manage access to care [12]. However, few studies have correlated the chances of undergoing CABG through unplanned emergency admission with the time spent on a CABG wait list after registration for elective surgery. In particular, there is little information on the chances of emergency surgery across priority groups. In addition, it is unclear whether expediting treatment reduces the number of unplanned emergency procedures in more urgent groups.

In Part II, Chapter 8, we summarize a study that aimed to describe the incidence of unplanned emergency surgery among patients waiting for isolated CABG and to determine whether shorter delays reduced the probability of emergency surgery among patients prioritized in more urgent groups. To estimate the time-dependent probability that a patient, who can be removed from the list through planned surgery, death, or other competing events, undergoes unplanned emergency surgery during or before a certain wait-list week, we prospectively analyzed actual waiting times from a population database of all patients registered for isolated CABG between 1991 and 2000 in British Columbia. To examine the relation between the length of delay and the cumulative incidence of emergency surgery, we first describe the probability of remaining on a waiting list by time since registration. Then, we compare the rate of emergency surgery per unit of wait-list time across priority groups using discrete-time survival models. Finally, we compare the cumulative incidence of emergency surgery across priority groups using competing-risks regression models for pseudovalues of cumulative incidence functions.

1.7.12 What is the relation between length of the wait list and chances of death while on the wait list?

The length of the wait list for surgery, a common correlate of the expected wait for hospital admission, is often the only information available to cardiologists and their patients in the decision where to seek surgical treatment. Indeed, all patients on a wait list must be treated before a patient who has just been registered for surgery can be scheduled for hospital admission. Surprisingly, few studies have correlated the health effects of the presurgical wait with wait-list size at the time of registration for elective cardiac surgery. It has been argued that cardiologists and their patients should assess the likely extent of treatment delay and associated risks when they choose a cardiac surgeon. The common concern is whether the decision to refer a patient to a specific cardiac surgeon can be made without considering the length of the current wait list.

1.7.13 What is the relation between length of the wait list and chances of unplanned emergency surgery?

Few studies have correlated the chances of undergoing unplanned emergency surgery from the wait list with wait-list size at the time of registration for elective surgery. However, this relation is important in deciding where to undergo treatment because wait-list size is often the only information available. The objective of a study we summarize in Part II, Chapter 8, was to compare the time-dependent probability of undergoing elective surgery through unplanned emergency admission between two groups of patients classified according to the length of wait lists at the time of registration for surgery. We also tested for significant differences in the risk of unplanned emergency surgery resulting from registration on a longer wait list.

1.7.14 What is the risk of death associated with delayed surgical treatment?

When reporting the mortality rate for patients who may die or undergo surgery, special statistical techniques must be used to isolate the effect of competing risks of surgery and death. The Kaplan-Meier method, which is used in randomized controlled trials of immediate CABG versus medical therapy, is not appropriate for describing the probability of competing outcomes over time [1]. Methodologically, not including preoperative deaths implies that survival time begins at the time of the procedure; therefore, treatment effect is implicitly conditional on surviving to treatment. The proportion of patients scheduled for CABG who die preoperatively is affected by the incidence of both surgery and death, and it is therefore unclear whether the low observed probabilities of death indicate a true low risk of death or appropriate timing of surgery.

One measure suggested for summarizing the risk of death over time in a setting of competing risks is the probability of death conditional on not having experienced the competing event by a certain time [73]. Using this approach, we sought to improve the estimates of the risk of death associated with delaying CABG among patients requiring the operation. We therefore estimated the time-dependent probability of death, given that CABG was not performed by certain times, using data from a prospective database of all adult patients who were accepted for isolated first-time CABG.

1.7.15 What is the survival benefit of coronary artery bypass grafting?

Randomized trials and observational studies have demonstrated survival benefits conferred by CABG [96]. The intervention has been shown to improve long-term survival in stable symptomatic patients with left main coronary artery disease, triple-vessel disease, or two-vessel disease with significant stenosis of the proximal left anterior descending coronary artery [122]. In practice, however, personal reasons, scheduling procedures, and surgical wait lists can delay CABG after a decision to operate has been made [36]. Hannan et al. argued that estimates of survival benefits conferred by CABG should account for the total number of deaths, including deaths resulting from delays for required revascularization [50]. We anticipate that such estimates can show the difference in the risk of death between patients who actually undergo required CABG and those who remain untreated after the decision to treat. The purpose of this analysis is to compare survival after the treatment decision in patients who undergo CABG and those who remain untreated. We used observational data from a population-based registry of patients with established coronary artery disease for whom surgical revascularization was indicated and planned.

1.8 Types of inferences

In health services research on access to care, we are mostly concerned with differences in proportions, rates, and distributions across periods, regions, procedures, or groups of patients. We would like to know whether the proportion of patients undergoing surgery within the target access time is similar for two calendar periods, whether the rate of admissions from wait lists for different procedures is the same, and whether waiting time becomes shorter when additional funds become available. In statistical terms, we must estimate the effects of factors interfering with access by describing odds ratios, rate ratios, and hazard ratios associated with categories of explanatory variables. We can further estimate the effects of those factors by expressing the probability of admission through a regression function of study variables.

1.9 Statistical challenges

The statistical challenges associated with analyzing waiting-time data include the question of how to address incomplete observations or unobserved heterogeneity between patients. Random-effects modeling of right-censored and left-truncated observations is the most useful analytical tool to address this issue [63]. Measured as the number of scheduling cycles, each providing a single opportunity for elective admission, time to admission is inherently discrete. Therefore, statistical analysis of waiting-time data could take advantage of discrete time-to-event models [2].

1.9.1 Incomplete observations

In studies of waiting times, the interest often lies in summarizing time since registration among patients who were registered for treatment sequentially in calendar time. As reported elsewhere [10, 103], ten percent of patients accepted for treatment can expect to be removed from the wait list, after spending some time on the list, for reasons other than receiving the treatment. Some of these patients may experience other competing events, such as health deterioration or emergency treatment. Other patients may decide against surgery or decline admission; some may move from the area and contact with them may be lost. In a prospective study, an observation for a patient removed from the list before admission occurs is considered incomplete; in this situation, the recorded waiting time is less than it otherwise would be. Observations may be also censored when the study is restricted by date, and only a portion of the waiting time is observable for patients registered near the end of the study period. If they are still on the list at the end of the study, their ultimate waiting times are unknown. These observations are said to be *right* censored, since all that is known is that time to admission exceeds the observed value.

This idea is explained by the Lexis diagram, which summarizes waiting times collected in a prospective study (Figure 1.1). In general, the Lexis diagram is a coordinate system with calendar time in the horizontal direction and follow-up time in the vertical direction. In Figure 1.1, slanted bars represent time courses for individual patients' waiting times, graphed in ascending order of registration date; the abscissa shows the date each patient was registered, u, and the ordinate shows the elapsed time since registration, v. Patient i enters the diagram at $(u, v) = (b_i, 0)$, wait-list week 0, and progresses week by week diagonally until (u_i, v_i), the last week on the list. The right end of the abscissa indicates the end of a study period at which observations for all patients remaining on the list are censored. By drawing a horizontal line at a specific waiting time, the magnitude of the risk set at that time and the amount of follow-up beyond it can be examined. For example, the bars crossed by the dashed line form the risk set of patients remaining on the wait lists at 52 weeks after registration for treatment.

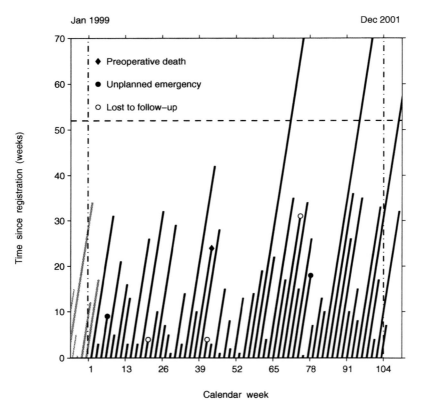

Fig. 1.1. Lexis diagram of waiting times. Each slanted bar is the time course of a single patient after registration on a wait list. A cohort study will use waiting-time data from all patients registered between January 1, 1991 and December 31, 2001 and followed up to the end of the study period. The gray bars indicate patients registered before the study period. The bars of patients remaining on the wait lists at the end of follow-up are censored. The bars crossed by the dashed line represent patients remaining on the wait lists at 52 weeks after registration for treatment.

Sometimes patients registered to a specialist's wait list are then referred to another specialist for additional investigations. If this referral results in a long delay, these patients are temporarily "put on hold" until they receive the specialist's approval for treatment. Observations for these patients are said to be *left* censored since all that is known is that time to admission is actually less than the interval between registration and admission, and part of that time was spent waiting for the investigation, not for treatment.

Regular regression analysis of waiting times cannot cope with the uncertainty in the data caused by censoring. However, censored observations should not be withdrawn from the analysis. If the censored observations are not accounted for, the estimated probabilities of receiving the service may be biased toward a higher rate, and the median and mean waiting time may be underestimated [104]. The methods of time-to-event analysis allow us to use incomplete information in a sample [66]. A fundamental assumption that makes use of these methods is that the distribution of censored time does not depend on the parameters governing waiting-times distribution. If, however, censoring were related to the mechanism governing admissions, this assumption would result in biased estimates of the probability of receiving the service within a certain time.

1.9.2 Truncated samples

Another challenging data feature is largely related to sampling schemes in which certain events or conditions may screen some patients from observation so that the investigator will not be aware of their existence. These samples must be considered *truncated*. The most common situation, *left* truncation, occurs when an event between acceptance and admission is used to identify individuals for a study. Sometimes it is a preceding procedure, a visit to a specialist, or the event of scheduling services. In this sampling scheme, patients removed from the list before these screening events take place will not be selected. Thus, the waiting experiences of such patients have no chance to contribute to the study. Here, the problem is not that the time from acceptance to admission is unavailable, but rather that patients must experience an intermediate event to be included in the study cohort. Therefore, observed waiting time should be greater than the smallest time from acceptance to an intermediate event. *Right* truncation arises in waiting-time studies that are based on the experience of those admitted, not those removed. Sampling consists of observing the waiting time within the observational window (0 to τ), usually fiscal year, or quarter, of registration. Only patients admitted for service before time τ are included in the sample. Admitted patients who have yet to be scheduled for the service are not included. Therefore, in addition to selection bias, patients who need longer waits are underrepresented.

1.9.3 Correlated observations

Several waiting times for the same patient might be considered as possibly correlated observations. For instance, in the aforementioned study on access to elective surgery, 11% of the patients accepted to surgery were added to the list two or three times [103]. Some patients had been reinstated on the list, whereas the others entered the list several times for different surgical procedures. Correlation between observations may cause some distortion in estimates and hypothesis testing. To address this problem, a model of the joint distribution of the two waiting times could be developed [100]. Alternatively, the model could be fitted using the generalized estimation equations [37].

1.9.4 Intermediate events

In prospective studies, information is often available on intermediate events that patients may experience between registration and admission to hospital for treatment. These include delay in scheduling the operation, cancellation of booked services, reinstatement following medical deferral, and failure to attend. The occurrence of the events preceding admission may alter the admission rate in one group and have no effect in the other, have the same effect in both groups, or have different effects in each group. The common concern is therefore potential bias in estimates of relative admission rates when a comparison does not take into account events preceding admission. Some argue that an adjustment should be made for time-varying variables when groups are compared [62]. The primary purpose of this adjustment is to see how the effects of the fixed factors change when intermediate events occur [67]. In addition, it may help to strengthen the inferences about how the intermediate event affects the admission rate [8].

Analysis of intermediate events raises some methodological complications. For instance, directly comparing patients who had a scheduling delay with patients who did not have such a delay may produce misleading results. First, patients from the first group must have stayed on a waiting list at least until the time of the event, whereas some patients in the second group might leave the list before the event occurs. Second, unlike main events, an intermediate event is not certain to occur; therefore, it is not appropriate to use the main event to censor intermediate events [69]. Measuring time to admission from the date of an intermediate event introduces bias toward a higher rate in the estimated probabilities of admission within a short duration of registration [10].

1.9.5 Competing risks

Competing risks naturally arise in wait-list settings. A competing event is "any event whose occurrence either precludes the occurrence of another event under examination or fundamentally alters the probability of occurrence of this other event" [45]. In the analysis of random durations, events are classified as competing events if their occurrence precludes the subsequent occurrence of the primary event or as censoring events if their occurrence precludes the observation but not the development of the primary event. For example, suppose the primary event of interest is death while on the wait list for surgery; then, undergoing the planned operation is a competing event, and loss to follow-up is a censoring event. A patient on a wait list is considered at risk of the primary event from time of registration until he or she experiences the primary event, a competing event, or a censoring event.

Waiting-time data used in this book

2.1 Patient progress through surgical care

Surgical care encompasses a continuum of activities through the diagnostic, preoperative, operative, and postoperative stages [28, 34]. During the diagnostic stage, the patient undergoes tests and other forms of evaluations to identify the condition causing illness, which may or may not require surgery. The preoperative stage consists of all the clinical and managerial activities that take place from when a decision to operate is taken until the patient enters the operating room. The operative stage lasts from the patient's entry into the operating room until his or her entry into the recovery suite. The postoperative stage includes recovery care and treatment in an inpatient surgical unit and/or an intensive care unit and ends with discharge from hospital.

The following is a summary of the processes in surgical care at major teaching hospitals in Canada. When necessary, primary care physicians refer to a specialist any patient who presents with signs and symptoms specific to a condition that is amenable to surgical intervention. If, following an outpatient consultation, surgery is deemed necessary, staff in the surgeon's office register the patient on an appropriate wait list and sends the request for operating room time to hospitals where the surgeon has admitting privileges. The patient is then scheduled for presurgical assessment at a preadmission clinic, where an anesthesiologist determines the patient's suitability for surgery and creates a care plan for the preoperative and postoperative periods [44]. The procedure is postponed if the patient is deemed unfit for any reason. If necessary, the patient undergoes additional preoperative investigations for assessment of surgical risks. Clinic staff provide education about the procedure and any preparation required at home.

Each patient's access to surgery is managed through the scheduling of operating room time [16]. Surgical scheduling staff identify the patients available for allocated operating room time slots and reserve hospital resources to ensure appropriate care during and after the operation [49]. Patients are selected for scheduling both from hospital wards and from the surgical wait lists on the basis of allocated operating room time slots.

Patients may be admitted to the hospital through the emergency room, the same-day admission clinic, or the patient admitting office. To allow optimal utilization of surgical suite resources, hospitals periodically release blocks of operating room time to various surgical services. Each service then places its patients on the operating room schedule, with some operative slots set aside for emergency cases [77]. Any time that is not booked by a particular service is then made available to other services. Each surgical service selects patients from its wait lists and schedules operations on the basis of urgency, best use of allocated operating time, availability of hospital resources, and plan for discharge from the hospital. Once set, the schedule for a particular service may be changed to accommodate the needs of emergency patients, who have preferential access to hospital resources. Conversely, scheduled surgery may be moved ahead if an operating room time slot becomes available.

On the day of a scheduled procedure, the anesthesiologist and the attending surgeon assess the patient before transfer to the operating room holding area. After the operation, the patient is taken to the postanesthesia care unit for monitoring and treatment of possible side effects of anesthesia. The anesthesiologist performs a postsurgical assessment, and the patient is transferred to the intensive care unit or to a hospital ward for further treatment [14].

While the patient is on the ward, a bedside nurse reassesses the patient's pain and other aspects of his or her condition. Once the patient reaches the point where oral analgesics are sufficient to control postsurgical pain, the primary surgical service takes over the task of following the patient. Finally, when the criteria for discharge are met, the patient is discharged from the hospital to home or to after-hospital care.

2.2 Access to coronary artery bypass grafting surgery

2.2.1 Capturing events in surgical cardiac care

In this section, we describe variables that reflect a patient's progress from the time of registration on a wait list for elective coronary artery bypass grafting (CABG) in British Columbia, Canada. Patients who are to undergo CABG may encounter different events along their individual care pathways. Figure 2.1 shows the care pathways and perioperative activities that patients presenting with symptoms of coronary artery disease are likely to experience, according to initial presentation and subsequent events leading to surgery. For example, a 55-year-old woman who is registered on a surgical wait list at a particular hospital may, at the time of registration, have an urgency status of semiurgent, with no comorbidities. Her subsequent care steps may involve a visit to the preadmission clinic, assessment by an anesthesiologist, the scheduled bypass surgery itself, and discharge from hospital. Alternatively, a 75-year-old man who is registered on a surgical wait list at a different hospital may, at the time of registration, have urgent status, with chronic obstructive pulmonary disease as a major comorbidity. If his condition deteriorates, his surgery may be cancelled because he is unfit to undergo the procedure. These various care pathways and characteristics of patients scheduled for CABG are captured through events and attributes of interest.

To reconstruct the events that patients experience during the perioperative period, health services researchers develop a data model that specifies the relations between data elements and events occurring during the process of care. In this book, data on patients who were registered to undergo CABG were obtained from the British Columbia Cardiac Registry (BCCR) [120]. This prospective database contains dates of registration on the list, procedure, and withdrawal from the list, along with disease severity and other risk factors, for all patients who have been registered to undergo CABG in any of the four tertiary care hospitals that provide cardiac care to adult residents of British Columbia since 1991 [110].

A time stamp is recorded for all captured events, so the time between events in the process of care is easily recovered. Therefore, we refer to patient-level information on events and their dates as waiting-time data. In the database that we used for our analysis, the sequence of events for individual patients can be presented in terms of patient-level records, whereby one patient has only one record with multiple variables representing the date and type of event, or by means of a patient-episode data set, in which each patient has multiple records. The patient-level format is best suited to presenting events that occur at regular intervals, in which case the fields containing event dates are labeled with numeric suffixes to relate the event date to the subsequent event [102]. For some factors that vary over time, an additional set of fields is needed to store information on the date and value of each factor. For example, if the hospital capacity changes quarterly,

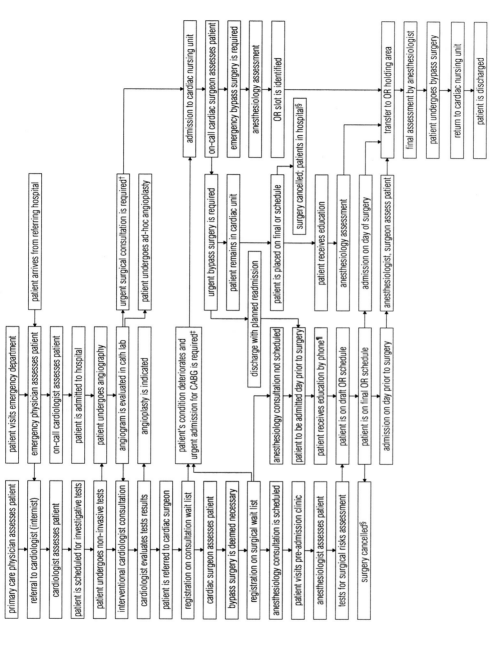

Fig. 2.1. Process of care for patients presenting with symptoms of coronary artery disease. Care coordinators †help to expedite surgical assessment, ‡contact patients at home until their procedures, §oversee re-scheduling of patients whose surgeries were cancelled, and ¶provide educational materials to patients and their families. (OR = operating room).

four additional variables are needed for 1 year of follow-up. In contrast, the person-episode record has for each patient only fields for event identification number and event date. The combination of patient identifier and sequential event number uniquely determines the record related to a certain event.

Registry records also provided information on each patient's age, sex, urgency status, coronary anatomy, and hospital at the time of registration on the wait list.

The primary events of interest for each patient were registration and removal from the wait list, hospital admission and separation, scheduled surgery and unplanned emergency surgery, and preoperative, in-hospital or follow-up death. The date of the surgeon's request to book the operating room served as the date of the decision for surgery and registration on a wait list. In British Columbia, surgical wait lists hold patient names until the surgery can be scheduled. Patients are removed from a wait list without surgery if they die, if they reconsider the decision to undergo surgery, if their condition deteriorates such that surgery is no longer possible, or if they undergo surgery elsewhere. Each week, the offices of all cardiac surgeons provide information to the registry on registrations for surgery, operations performed, wait-list reconciliation (removals), and discharge summaries.

2.2.2 Other data sources

Additional information on access to CABG was obtained from administrative health databases and provincial death records. To identify hospital admission and discharge dates, coexisting conditions, and whether the patient was discharged alive or died in hospital, we used each patient's provincial health number to link deterministically BCCR records to the British Columbia Linked Health Database Hospital Separations File. [25]. Data on coexisting conditions were retrieved in the form of diagnoses reported in discharge abstracts created during the calendar year before the treatment decision [56]. Unplanned emergency surgeries were identified by the emergent or urgent code for admission from the emergency department or by the emergent code for admission from the admitting department after the patient was registered on a surgical wait list. To identify deaths that did not occur in a hospital, we linked the BCCR to the British Columbia Linked Health Database Deaths File [117]. Underlying causes of death were coded according to the International Classification of Diseases, 9th revision (ICD-9). Deaths related to cardiovascular disease were represented by ICD-9 codes 410 to 414 (ischemic heart disease) or 420 to 429 (other forms of heart disease) [23].

2.2.3 Analytical data set

The registry records were linked to the other databases to create the analytical data set for patients registered for elective CABG. A data dictionary was created to describe the variables representing events and attributes of interest in this data set (Table 2.1). In this table, the rows show variables in the data set and the columns show characteristics of each variable, such as the name, the information stored in the variable, the data sources, the type of data, and how the data are coded. For example, the variable named "SEXF" contains data on the patient's sex and is a categorical variable where 0 indicates man and 1 indicates woman.

Table 2.1. Data dictionary for records of patients awaiting elective coronary bypass grafting

Variable	Description	Source	Code
BCCR_ID	Patient identifier	BCCR	\<Text\>
AGECAT	Age decade	BCCR	1 – 20–29 years
			2 – 30–39 years
			...
			8 – ≥90 years
SEXF	Sex	BCCR	0 – Man
			1 – Woman
ANATOM	Coronary anatomy	BCCR	1 – Left main disease
			2 – 2- or 3-vessel disease, with PLAD
			3 – 3-vessel disease, with no PLAD
			4 – 1-vessel disease, with PLAD
			5 – 1- or 2-vessel disease, no PLAD
			U – Otherwise and unknown
UR_BK	Urgency at booking	BCCR	0 – Emergency
			1 – Urgent
			2 – Semiurgent
			3 – Nonurgent
			U – Unknown
CM_CH	Comorbidities from Charlson index	Hospital Separations	0, 1, 2, 3, or 4 (≥4)
CM_BK	Major comorbidities	Hospital Separations	1 – CHF or diabetes or COPD or rheumatism or cancer
			0 – Other
INST_BK	Location at registration	BCCR	Hospital 1, 2, 3, or 4
WL_ST	Wait-list registration date	BCCR	mm/dd/yyyy
WL_EN	Wait-list removal date	BCCR	mm/dd/yyyy
WL_RM	Reason for removal	BCCR	0 – Underwent surgery
			1 – Death
			2 – Medical treatment
			3 – At patient request
			4 – Transfer to other hospital
			5 – Otherwise removed from list

			6 – No surgical report
			7 – Still on wait list
			8 – Other surgery
			9 – Death recorded in BCCR,
			not in Deaths File
DTHDATE	Death date	Deaths File	mm/dd/yyyy
			< . > – no date recorded
EXIT_CODE	Type of hospital discharge	Hospital Separations	D – Discharged alive
			S – Left against medical advice
			X – Died in hospital
			N/A – Not applicable
ADDATE	Hospital admission date	Hospital Separations	mm/dd/yyyy
			< . > – no date recorded
SEPDATE	Hospital separation date	Hospital Separations	mm/dd/yyyy
			< . > – no date recorded

Abbreviations: BCCR = British Columbia Cardiac Registry, CHF = congestive heart failure, COPD = chronic obstructive pulmonary disease, PLAD = proximal left anterior descending

Table 2.2 shows a sample of fictitious records from the analytical data set, in which each row represents a patient record and each column is a variable representing an event or attribute of interest. From each patient record, we can reconstruct the key events and attributes of the patient's care pathway. For example, patient 100002 was a man between 50 and 59 years of age, who had three-vessel disease with no proximal left anterior descending, and no comorbidities. On July 22, 1994, he was registered on a wait list for hospital 4, with semiurgent status. He was admitted to hospital on February 14, 1995; he underwent surgery and was removed from the wait list on February 17, 1995. He was discharged alive on February 27, 1995; however, he died on July 15, 1996.

2.2.4 Patient population

In Part II of this book, we present the results of several modeling studies that we performed using the records of patients for whom surgical revascularization was indicated at the time of consultation with a cardiac surgeon.

In British Columbia, there are two pathways to surgical revascularization: registration on a wait list or direct admission after coronary angiography. A patient who presents with symptoms of coronary artery disease is referred to a cardiologist, who evaluates the results of coronary angiography and recommends treatment. If coronary angioplasty is not indicated, the patient is referred to a cardiac surgeon, who assesses the need and suitability for CABG. Following the decision to operate, surgeons register on their wait lists patients who require and decide to undergo the operation.

Between January 1991 and December 2000, 9346 patients were registered for first-time isolated (without a valve-replacement procedure) CABG on the elective basis. We excluded the records of 147 patients for a variety of reasons: case was coded as an emergency at the time of registration (30 patients), patient was

Table 2.2. Sample of analytical data set for fictitious patients awaiting elective coronary artery bypass grafting

BCCR_ID	AGECAT	SEXF	ANATOM	UR_BK	CM_CH	CM_BK	INST_BK	WL_ST	WL_EN	WL_RM	DTHDATE	EXIT_CODE	ADDATE	SEPDATE
100001	5	0	1	2	0	0	2	01/29/1992	03/25/1992	0	.	D	03/24/1992	04/03/1992
100002	4	0	3	2	0	0	4	07/22/1994	02/17/1995	0	07/15/1996	D	02/14/1995	02/27/1995
100003	4	1	3	1	2	0	2	08/23/1996	08/24/1996	0	.	D	08/23/1996	09/01/1996
100004	3	0	3	3	0	0	3	09/17/1991	11/08/1991	0	.	D	11/07/1991	11/13/1991
100005	7	0	1	2	3	1	2	07/13/1997	10/24/1997	0	.	D	10/25/1997	11/09/1997
100006	4	0	3	2	2	1	2	04/21/1993	06/05/1993	0	06/15/1993	X	06/05/1993	06/10/1993
100007	5	1	3	2	4	1	2	10/09/1995	01/23/1996	1	01/15/1996	N/A	.	.
100008	6	0	3	3	3	1	1	02/20/1998	03/13/1998	2	.	N/A	.	.
100009	3	0	5	2	0	0	4	11/22/1992	12/31/1992	5	.	N/A	.	.
100010	4	0	3	2	0	0	2	12/04/1996	01/16/1997	5	03/15/2001	N/A	.	.

removed from the list on the registration date (99), operating room report was missing (4), or registration on a weekend with admission the next day, which suggests immediate access (14). The records for the remaining 9199 patients (see Table 2.3 for baseline characteristics) had either a surgery date or a date of removal without surgery (and a reason for this event). The study period ended in December 2001, which allowed only 52 weeks of follow-up after the last patients were added to the list. Therefore, we restricted the analysis to the first 52 weeks after registration, such that the 471 patients (5.1%) remaining on the lists at 12 months were censored. Of those, 167 eventually underwent surgery, 7 died, 78 became unfit for surgery, 187 declined surgery, 16 were transferred to another surgeon or hospital, and 99 were removed from the wait lists for other reasons. Among the 8728 patients (94.9%) who were removed from the list by 52 weeks, 7654 received planned surgery, 314 underwent unplanned emergency surgery, 91 died, 173 became unfit for surgery, 104 declined surgery, 98 were transferred to another surgeon or hospital, 23 received other surgery, and 188 were removed for other reasons.

Alternatively, when urgent assessment is deemed necessary, patients are admitted to a hospital cardiac ward directly from the catheterization laboratory. If suitable for surgery, such patients remain in hospital until the operation. There were 10 467 direct admissions between January 1991 and December 2001 (see Table 2.4 for baseline characteristics). The data dictionary for the analytical data set of directly admitted CABG patients is shown in the Appendix (Table A.1).

To prioritize patients and assign the target access time for surgery, all cardiac surgeons in British Columbia used established guidelines developed in 1990, which was based on the severity of angina symptoms, the extent of coronary artery disease (including the extent of left main stenosis), the results of noninvasive tests, and the presence of left ventricular dysfunction (ejection fraction less than 50%) as described elsewhere [70]. There were three priority groups at registration for CABG: urgent, semiurgent, and nonurgent. The target time to surgery was 3 days for patients with left main coronary artery stenosis greater than 70% (urgent group); 6 weeks for patients with persistent unstable angina, impaired left ventricular function, and significant obstruction, defined as left-main stenosis, triple-vessel disease, or double-vessel disease with significant stenosis of the proximal left anterior descending artery (semiurgent group); and 12 weeks for patients with intractable chronic angina, normal left ventricular function, and single-vessel disease or double-vessel disease with no lesion in the proximal left anterior descending artery (nonurgent group).

2.3 Access to elective vascular surgery

2.3.1 Data sources

Data were obtained from a hospital registry set up by the Department of Surgery, Queen's University, Kingston, Ontario, to prospectively collect data on waiting times for admission of patients registered for elective vascular surgery. The registry records accounted for all patients referred to the department for assessment at the outpatient clinic who were afterward added to the wait list. Patients who received emergency treatment were excluded. The data dictionary for the vascular data, which describes variables representing events and attributes of interest, appears in Table A.2.

2.3.2 Patient population

We studied the records of patients for whom elective vascular surgery was indicated and planned. Patients were registered on the wait list after the consultation visit during which surgery was deemed necessary.

Table 2.3. Characteristics of 9199 patients registered for elective isolated coronary artery bypass grafting in British Columbia, 1991–2000

	Priority group; no. (%) of patients			
Characteristic	All* (n = 9199)	Urgent (n = 646)	Semiurgent (n = 6481)	Nonurgent (n = 1959)
Age group (years)				
<50	731 (7.9)	37 (5.7)	497 (7.7)	187 (9.5)
50–59	2002 (21.8)	128 (19.8)	1404 (21.7)	452 (23.1)
60–69	3511 (38.2)	250 (38.7)	2491 (38.4)	728 (37.2)
70–79	2763 (30.0)	207 (32.0)	1963 (30.3)	554 (28.3)
≥80	192 (2.1)	24 (3.7)	126 (1.9)	38 (1.9)
Registration period				
1991–1992	1723 (18.7)	116 (18.0)	1220 (18.8)	334 (17.0)
1993–1994	1883 (20.5)	110 (17.0)	1377 (21.2)	386 (19.7)
1995–1996	1995 (21.7)	237 (36.7)	1360 (21.0)	374 (19.1)
1997–1998	1884 (20.5)	116 (18.0)	1324 (20.4)	428 (21.8)
1999–2000	1714 (18.6)	67 (10.4)	1200 (18.5)	437 (22.3)
Sex				
Men	7572 (82.3)	526 (81.4)	5365 (82.8)	1581 (80.7)
Women	1627 (17.7)	120 (18.6)	1116 (17.2)	378 (19.3)
Comorbidity at registration				
Major conditions[†]	2004 (21.8)	163 (25.2)	1391 (21.5)	424 (21.6)
Other conditions[‡]	2431 (26.4)	217 (33.6)	1765 (27.2)	421 (21.5)
None	4764 (51.8)	266 (41.2)	3325 (51.3)	1114 (56.9)
Location at registration				
Hospital 1	1895 (20.6)	130 (20.1)	1371 (21.2)	385 (19.7)
Hospital 2	3130 (34.0)	282 (43.7)	2467 (38.1)	371 (18.9)
Hospital 3	2121 (23.1)	18 (2.8)	1022 (15.8)	1019 (52.0)
Hospital 4	2053 (22.3)	216 (33.4)	1621 (25.0)	184 (9.4)
Coronary anatomy				
Left main disease	1411 (15.3)	401 (62.1)	972 (15.0)	32 (1.6)
Multivessel[§]	7025 (76.4)	215 (33.3)	5075 (78.3)	1692 (86.4)
Limited[‖]	763 (8.3)	30 (4.6)	434 (6.7)	235 (12.0)

* Includes 113 patients with unknown priority group

[†] Congestive heart failure, diabetes mellitus, chronic obstructive pulmonary disease, rheumatoid arthritis, or cancer

[‡] Peripheral vascular disease, cerebrovascular disease, dementia, peptic ulcer disease, hemiplegia, renal disease, or liver disease

[§] Two- or three-vessel disease with proximal left anterior descending (PLAD)

[‖] Two-vessel disease with no PLAD or one-vessel disease with PLAD

Table 2.4. Characteristics of 10 467 direct admissions for isolated coronary artery bypass grafting in British Columbia, 1991–2001

Characteristic	Priority group; no. (%) of patients			
	All* (*n* = 10467)	Urgent (*n* = 5353)	Semiurgent (*n* = 4536)	Nonurgent (*n* = 523)
Age group (years)				
<50	808 (7.7)	384 (7.2)	374 (8.2)	46 (8.8)
50–59	2082 (19.9)	1040 (19.4)	910 (20.1)	126 (24.1)
60–69	3689 (35.2)	1851 (34.6)	1616 (35.6)	198 (37.9)
70–79	3509 (33.5)	1856 (34.7)	1493 (32.9)	141 (27.0)
≥80	379 (3.6)	222 (4.1)	143 (3.2)	12 (2.3)
Surgery period				
1991–1992	1770 (16.9)	777 (14.5)	826 (18.2)	152 (29.1)
1993–1994	1526 (14.6)	985 (18.4)	503 (11.1)	37 (7.1)
1995–1996	1686 (16.1)	1004 (18.8)	600 (13.2)	82 (15.7)
1997–1998	1997 (19.1)	1044 (19.5)	856 (18.9)	86 (16.4)
1999–2000	2454 (23.4)	1081 (20.2)	1199 (26.4)	156 (29.8)
2001	1034 (9.9)	462 (8.6)	552 (12.2)	10 (1.9)
Sex				
Men	8154 (77.9)	4059 (75.8)	3603 (79.4)	441 (84.3)
Women	2313 (22.1)	1294 (24.2)	933 (20.6)	82 (15.7)
Comorbidity at surgery				
Major conditions[†]	4040 (38.6)	2046 (38.2)	1803 (39.7)	171 (32.7)
Other conditions[‡]	5268 (50.3)	2853 (53.3)	2221 (49.0)	170 (32.5)
None	1159 (11.1)	454 (8.5)	512 (11.3)	182 (34.8)
Location at surgery				
Hospital 1	1590 (15.2)	558 (10.4)	1007 (22.2)	20 (3.8)
Hospital 2	2522 (24.1)	1500 (28.0)	920 (20.3)	101 (19.3)
Hospital 3	4362 (41.7)	2149 (40.1)	1811 (39.9)	364 (69.6)
Hospital 4	1993 (19.0)	1146 (21.4)	798 (17.6)	38 (7.3)

* Includes 55 patients with unknown priority group

[†] Congestive heart failure, diabetes mellitus, chronic obstructive pulmonary disease, rheumatoid arthritis, or cancer

[‡] Peripheral vascular disease, cerebrovascular disease, dementia, peptic ulcer disease, hemiplegia, renal disease, or liver disease

Patients were removed from the list if they reconsidered their decision for surgery, if they died while await-ing surgery, if their condition deteriorated so that the operation was no longer possible, if their condition improved and the surgery therefore became unnecessary, or when surgery was performed.

All 1916 adult cases registered for elective vascular surgery between July 1994 and March 2002 were followed until surgery, until removal from the wait list without surgery, or December 31, 2002. Altogether, 1845 patients (96.3%) were removed from the list within 40 weeks of registration. The remainder had waits longer than 40 weeks: for 18 patients, surgery was deferred indefinitely by the surgeon; 7 patients declined planned surgery; the condition of 4 patients improved; 1 patient died; and 41 patients whose procedures had been initially deferred (24 at the physician's request and 17 at the patient's request) eventually had surgery. Missing information made it impossible to adjust these extended waits for periods when surgery could not be performed. Therefore, we restricted our analysis to the first 40 weeks of follow-up and considered these 71 observations to have been censored at 40 weeks. Of the total number of patients registered, 1743 (91.0%) underwent surgery, 71 (3.7%) were still waiting at 40 weeks, and 102 (5.3%) were removed from the list without surgery for various reasons: the patient's condition improved (23), the patient died while awaiting surgery (5), the surgical risk became too great (57), or the patient decided against surgery (17).

2.3.3 Priority groups

In vascular surgery, the urgency of the patient's need for an intervention can be clearly defined. Clinical urgency status, assigned on the basis of the patient's condition, defines the maximum allowable delay before the procedure takes place. As described elsewhere [106], an internal protocol in the Department of Surgery was used to determine the number of days that a patient can safely wait for the planned operation according to clinical urgency. However, a previous analysis showed wide variations in individual waits among patients with equal need and clinical urgency [103]. In that study, we found that for some surgical procedures pa-tients with less urgent status had a chance of being admitted before patients with more urgent status. Patient- or hospital-related delays in scheduling surgery have been suggested as an explanation. For example, can-cellations of booked surgery may lengthen waiting periods independent of the urgency status assigned at registration. We therefore based our analysis on queuing patterns observed in practice, rather than urgency status assigned at registration. Queuing priority groups were defined as shown in Table 2.5, with smaller numbers indicating higher priority.

2.4 Access to elective cholecystectomy

2.4.1 Data sources

At the time of our study, the Department of Surgery at Queen's University was housed in two tertiary refer-ral centers providing services to more than half a million residents of southeastern Ontario. Eight general surgeons were performing cholecystectomy at that time. Each surgeon's office operated its own wait list independently, and there was no priority ranking system. Surgeons on call made the decision to operate on patients who presented to the emergency department by evaluating (a) the clinical presentation for symptoms and signs of persistent or worsening abdominal tenderness, guarding, or rebound; (b) the ultrasonographic finding of a thick-walled gallbladder with pericholecystic fluid or a finding of hepatobilary iminodiacetic acid on radionuclide scan; or (c) both (a) and (b).

Data on the timing and type of surgery were retrieved from the hospital's electronic patient information system. Information on the date of the consultation visit was obtained from patient records through the

Table 2.5. Characteristics of 1916 patients registered for elective vascular surgery in Ontario, 1994–2002

	Priority status*; no. (%) of patients				
	1	**2**	**3**	**4**	**5**
Characteristic	**(n = 344)**	**(n = 149)**	**(n = 247)**	**(n = 313)**	**(n = 863)**
Age group (years)					
<45	2 (0.6)	0 (0.0)	3 (1.2)	0 (0.0)	105 (12.2)
45–64	83 (24.1)	22 (14.8)	60 (24.3)	60 (19.2)	293 (34.0)
65–74	137 (39.8)	63 (42.3)	112 (45.3)	158 (50.5)	287 (33.3)
≥75	122 (35.5)	64 (43.0)	72 (29.1)	95 (30.4)	178 (20.6)
Registration period					
1994–1996	232 (67.4)	89 (59.7)	167 (67.6)	189 (60.4)	629 (72.9)
1997–2002	112 (32.6)	60 (40.3)	80 (32.4)	124 (39.6)	234 (27.1)
Sex					
Men	219 (63.7)	116 (77.9)	144 (58.3)	250 (79.9)	510 (59.1)
Women	125 (36.3)	33 (22.1)	103 (41.7)	63 (20.1)	353 (40.9)
Procedure					
AAA repair	23 (6.7)	149 (100.0)	0 (0.0)	313 (100.0)	0 (0.0)
CEA	0 (0.0)	0 (0.0)	247 (100.0)	0 (0.0)	164 (19.0)
PVD surgery	321 (93.3)	0 (0.0)	0 (0.0)	0 (0.0)	331 (38.4)
AVF	0 (0.0)	0 (0.0)	0 (0.0)	0 (0.0)	368 (42.6)

Abbreviations: AAA = abdominal aortic aneurysm, CEA = carotid endarterectomy,

PVD = peripheral vascular disease, AVF = arteriovenous fistula

* Lower numbers indicate greater priority

quality assurance program of the Department of Surgery. Patients who underwent emergency surgery without a prior clinic appointment were excluded. All cholecystectomies were initially attempted as laparoscopic procedures. Conversion to the open procedure was required when the dissection was not technically feasible or safe. The data dictionary for the cholecystectomy data, which describes variables representing events and attributes of interest, appears in Table A.3.

2.4.2 Patient population

We identified, for the period 1997 to 2000, all adult patients who underwent emergency or elective cholecystectomy after being seen in clinic for biliary colic. Forty-one of the patients were excluded from the analysis because they had immediate access (within 3 days) to planned surgery, which left a sample of 761 patients (Table 2.6).

Table 2.6. Characteristics of 761 patients registered for cholecystectomy in Ontario, 1997–2000

| | No. (%) of patients | | |
| | All cases | Elective | Emergency |
Characteristic	($n = 761$)	($n = 710$)	($n = 51$)
Age group (years)			
<25	33 (4.3)	28 (3.9)	5 (9.8)
25–34	105 (13.8)	98 (13.8)	7 (13.7)
35–44	142 (18.7)	138 (19.4)	4 (7.8)
45–54	170 (22.3)	161 (22.7)	9 (17.6)
55–64	155 (20.4)	148 (20.8)	7 (13.7)
65–74	107 (14.1)	97 (13.7)	10 (19.6)
≥75	49 (6.4)	40 (5.6)	9 (17.6)
Sex			
Men	189 (24.8)	179 (25.2)	10 (19.6)
Women	572 (75.2)	531 (74.8)	41 (80.4)
Registration period			
1997–1998	282 (37.1)	263 (37.0)	19 (37.3)
1998–1999	270 (35.5)	254 (35.8)	16 (31.4)
1999–2000	209 (27.5)	193 (27.2)	16 (31.4)
Surgeon's annual case volume			
<20	54 (7.1)	34 (4.8)	20 (39.2)
20–40	292 (38.4)	278 (39.2)	14 (27.5)
>40	415 (54.5)	398 (56.1)	17 (33.3)

Waits and outcomes: What should be reported?

3.1 Introduction

This chapter presents statistical methods for the analysis of waiting-time data. In section 3.2 we introduce descriptive statistics that are used to summarize the frequency of events on wait lists. We provide the definition, estimation procedure, and interpretation for each summary measure, such as proportions, rates, cumulative incidence function. Measures of comparison and corresponding tests for comparing these measures statistically across groups are presented in section 3.3. Finally, section 3.4 describes regression models that are used to quantify the effects of explanatory variables on wait-list outcomes. For each model we show how to interpret the regression coefficients based on concepts from the previous two sections.

3.2 Descriptive statistics

3.2.1 Notation

Consider a wait-list population exposed to two competing risks, for example surgery, and death before surgery. Let event 1 be the primary event of interest and event 2 the competing event, and let T_m denote the latent time to event $m = 1, 2$. In this competing-risks setting, we observe the time to removal from the list $T = \min\{T_1, T_2\}$ and the cause for removal $\delta = \text{argmin}_m\{T_m\}$. If neither event occurs during the study period or the patient is lost to follow-up, the observation is considered censored at the time of removal from the wait list or the end of follow-up. Censored observations are included in the vector of observed times. The joint distribution of the random variables (T, δ) is of interest, where it is not assumed that the competing risks act independently.

Suppose the events occur at E distinct, unevenly spaced, ordered times $t_1, t_2, \ldots, t_E$, and define $t_0 = 0$. Without loss of generality, we assume that time is measured in calendar weeks. Using Gooley's notation, let e_i be the number of primary events at time t_i, r_i be the number of competing events at time t_i, c_i be the number of censored events at time t_i, and $n_i = n_{i-1} - (e_i + r_i + c_i)$ be the number of patients still waiting beyond time t_i, where n_0 is the initial number of patients at risk [45].

We use this notation throughout this section. Although we consider only two types of events, the primary event and the competing event, events other than the primary event may be combined into the risk of a single competing event [91].

3.2.2 Proportions and odds

Definition

Proportions summarize the fraction of patients who experience a certain event. For instance, the weekly proportion of patients who were admitted, the proportion of patients who underwent surgery within target access times (TAT), and the proportion of patients who died before surgery are important indicators used to characterize access to elective surgery [114, 115, 116].

Although the proportion is the common measure for the probability of an event, an alternative is the odds of the event, which is defined as the ratio of the expected number of times that the event will occur to the expected number of times it will not occur [4]. For instance, the odds of death on the wait list by 52 weeks may be of interest. Unlike proportions, which are bounded by 0 and 1, the odds have a lower limit of 0 but no upper limit.

Estimation

To estimate the event proportion among waiting patients, p, the number of events observed is divided by the total number of patients at risk:

$$\hat{p} = \frac{\text{total number of events observed}}{\text{total number of patients at risk}}. \tag{3.1}$$

For example, the estimated proportion of patients who were admitted for surgery during week i from the time of their registration on a wait list is estimated as

$$\hat{p}_i = \frac{e_i}{n_{i-1}}. \tag{3.2}$$

In this example, the event is surgery during week i, and the patients at risk are those who were still on the wait list at the beginning of that week.

Another example is the proportion of patients who underwent surgery within the TAT, which is estimated by

$$\hat{p} = \frac{1}{n_0} \sum_{\{i|t_i \leq \text{TAT}\}} e_i. \tag{3.3}$$

Here, the event of interest is surgery within the TAT from registration, and the patients at risk are all those accepted on a wait list.

Similar quantities can be defined for events competing with the occurrence of surgery. The estimated proportion of patients who experienced the competing event, say preoperative death, within 52 weeks of registration is

$$\hat{p} = \frac{1}{n_0} \sum_{\{i|t_i \leq 52 \text{ weeks}\}} r_i. \tag{3.4}$$

In this example, the event of interest is death on the wait list within 52 weeks from registration, and the patients at risk are all those accepted for surgery.

For large sample sizes, one can use the normal approximation to the binomial distribution to obtain approximate $100(1 - \alpha)\%$ confidence intervals (CI) for the sample proportion $\hat{p}$ given by the following formula

$$\hat{p} \pm z_{1-\alpha/2} \sqrt{\hat{p}(1 - \hat{p})/n} \,, \tag{3.5}$$

where $z_{1-\alpha/2}$ is the $100(1 - \alpha/2)$th quantile of the standard normal distribution, n is the number of patients at risk, and $\sqrt{\hat{p}(1 - \hat{p})/n}$ is the standard error of the estimated proportion $\hat{p}$ [29]. For a 95% CI, $\alpha = 0.05$ and $z_{0.975} = 1.96$.

The estimated odds of an event is simply the ratio of the estimated proportion of the event to its complement [74]:

$$\widehat{\text{odds}} = \frac{\hat{p}}{1 - \hat{p}} \,. \tag{3.6}$$

Interpretation

By multiplying the proportion by 100, one can estimate the expected number of events among 100 patients on the list. Alternatively, the resulting quantity can be interpreted as the percentage of patients experiencing the event. In Part II of this volume, we use proportions for analysis of surgical waiting times. For instance, the weekly proportions of admissions by week and priority group are shown in Figure 5.3. The estimated percentage of nonurgent patients who underwent surgery within 12 weeks from the time of their registration for elective coronary artery bypass grafting (CABG) was 27.7% (95% CI 25.8–29.7) (Table 7.1). The estimated percentage of patients who died on the wait list within 52 weeks from registration for elective CABG was 1.0% (95% CI 0.8–1.2) (Table 8.2).

The odds of 1 imply that the presence of the event is just as likely as its absence. Similarly, odds less than 1 imply that the absence of the event is more likely and odds greater than 1 imply that the presence of the event is more likely. For example, the odds of 2 mean that the event is twice as likely to occur as to not occur. In Part II, we estimated the odds that a patient awaiting elective CABG dies on the wait list by 52 weeks as 0.01 (0.01/0.99). Thus, the expected number of deaths on the wait list is one-hundredth the number of survivals. Note that in the case of a rare event, such as death on the wait list, the estimated odds is close to the estimated proportion.

Remarks

Proportions are informative statistics for summarizing events among patients. However, they do not account for the time that patients spend on wait lists. In the next section, we describe event rates as an alternative summary measure which accounts for waiting time.

For the $100(1 - \alpha)\%$ CI of $\hat{p}$ in equation 3.5, it is possible for the confidence limits to lie below 0 or exceed 1. Generally, one should use a continuity correction if $n\hat{p}$ or $n(1 - \hat{p})$ are not well above 5. For small sample sizes, an exact confidence interval may be derived from the binomial distribution [29].

3.2.3 Hazard and rates

Definition

For a continuous time t, the event-specific hazard,

$$\lambda_m(t) = \lim_{h \to 0} \frac{\Pr(t \le T < t+h, \delta = m | T > t)}{h} , \qquad (3.7)$$

represents the instantaneous probability of event m at time t, conditional on remaining at risk of the event by time t. For discrete times $t_1, t_2, \ldots$, say weeks since registration for surgery, the event-specific hazard is defined as

$$\lambda_m(t_i) = \Pr(T = t_i | T \ge t_i) , \qquad (3.8)$$

which is the probability that event m occurs in a certain week t_i, conditional on remaining on the list until that week.

For discrete times, the cumulative hazard function of time,

$$\Lambda_m(t) = \sum_{\{i | t_i \le t\}} \lambda_m(t_i) , \qquad (3.9)$$

characterizes the risk of event m accumulated over a certain time t when competing risks are removed [66].

In health services research, the cumulative hazard is predominantly interpreted as the population mean number of events occurring by time t

$$\Lambda(t) = E\{N(t)\} ,$$

where $N(t)$ is a random variable counting the occurrence of the event over time t. The $\Lambda(t)$ is a function of time, therefore its derivative

$$\lambda(t) = \frac{d}{dt} \Lambda(t)$$

is interpreted as the event rate function.

When the event rate changes with time, it summarizes the frequency of events in a time interval of one-unit length [2], say the weekly rate of admission when observed times, t_i, are measured in weeks. When the event rate is constant over the length of the study period, $\lambda(t) = \lambda$, it summarizes the frequency of events experienced by patients accounting for the total amount of time that patients were at risk of the event, which is known as patient-time at risk. For instance, the number of weeks that all patients spent on the wait list is the sum of the number of weeks for each patient. The expected number of events by time t when event rate λ is constant is given by

$$\Lambda(t) = \lambda \times t , \qquad (3.10)$$

which for example gives the number of preoperative deaths occurring by 52 weeks after registration on surgical wait lists in a region that reports a certain death rate.

Estimation

The Nelson–Aalen estimator for the cumulative hazard function of the competing event, that is, $m = 2$, is

$$\hat{\Lambda}_2(t) = \sum_{\{i | t_i \le t\}} \frac{r_i}{n_{i-1}} , \qquad (3.11)$$

where $\frac{r_i}{n_{i-1}}$ is an estimate of the rate of the competing event $\lambda_2(t_i)$. The estimated variance of the Nelson–Aalen estimator is [66]

$$\widehat{\mathrm{Var}}(\hat{\Lambda}_2(t)) = \sum_{\{i|t_i \leq t\}} \frac{r_i}{(n_{i-1})^2} \, . \tag{3.12}$$

Alternatively, if the competing-event rate is estimated as an average over the length of the study period, $\overline{\lambda}_2$, then the cumulative hazard function is estimated by

$$\tilde{\Lambda}_2(t) = \overline{\lambda}_2 \times t \, . \tag{3.13}$$

To calculate the average event rate among waiting patients, the number of events is divided by the total patient-time spent on the list [52]:

$$\overline{\lambda}_m = \frac{\text{total number of type } m \text{ events observed}}{\text{total waiting time}} \, . \tag{3.14}$$

The denominator represents the total waiting time that all patients have contributed to the study [29]. In Gooley's notation, the estimated average weekly competing-event rate is

$$\overline{\lambda}_2 = \sum_{i=0}^{E} \frac{r_i}{t_i(e_i + r_i + c_i)} \, , \tag{3.15}$$

with estimated variance [52]

$$\widehat{\mathrm{Var}}(\overline{\lambda}_2) = \frac{(\overline{\lambda}_2)^2}{\sum_{i=0}^{E} r_i} \, . \tag{3.16}$$

Therefore, an approximate $100(1-\alpha)\%$ CI for the average competing-event rate is

$$\overline{\lambda}_2 \pm z_{1-\alpha/2} \sqrt{\widehat{\mathrm{Var}}(\overline{\lambda}_2)} \, , \tag{3.17}$$

where $z_{1-\alpha/2}$ is the $100(1-\alpha/2)$th quantile of the standard normal distribution. For a 95% CI, $\alpha = 0.05$ and $z_{0.975} = 1.96$.

Interpretation

When event rates are small, it is convenient to scale the rates. For example, multiplying a surgery rate of 0.097 per patient per week by 100 allows the rate to be expressed as 9.7 per 100 patient-weeks. The latter may be more readily interpreted as almost 10 surgeries expected for every 100 patient-weeks on average. In Part II, the average weekly death rate among all patients awaiting elective CABG is reported as 0.67 (95% CI 0.53–0.80) per 1000 patient-weeks (Table 8.1), which we interpret as almost 1 preoperative death per every 1000 weeks of the total waiting time. Among semiurgent and nonurgent patients who register to undergo CABG, the cumulative hazard was approximately linear with time spent on wait lists (Figure 8.2). Among these patients, the average weekly death rate was 0.00061 per patient-week. Therefore, by 52 weeks on the list, 3 deaths would be expected for every 100 patients placed on the wait lists ($0.00061 \times 52 = 0.03$).

Remarks

The cumulative hazard and event rates are useful statistics for summarizing events among patients who are on wait lists for different lengths of time. For example, the admission rate, which is the conditional probability of leaving the wait list for service in a certain week, represents the average proportion of patients admitted from a wait list. Unlike the proportions that we discussed in the previous section, the event rates account for the amount of time that patients spend on wait lists, by adjusting the at-risk set at the beginning of consecutive weeks.

Although accurately describing the instantaneous risk of an event, event-specific rates cannot be converted into the probabilities of events without the unrealistic and unverifiable assumption that time to primary event and time to competing event are independent [45].

Despite that it is always possible to calculate an average event rate over the study period, such an average rate may not be representative if the rate varies during the period. In this case, the study period should be divided into adjacent intervals and the interval-specific rate calculated. To determine if the risk of an event varies with the duration of the wait, the rate can be calculated for intervals of time on the wait list.

A constant event rate or exponentially distributed waiting times are required to obtain reasonable summaries of average event-specific rates [52]. The slope of the estimated event-specific cumulative hazard in equation 3.11 provides crude estimates of the event rate [66]. If the cumulative hazard is linearly related to the time spent on the wait list, then a constant rate is implied.

For the $100(1-\alpha)\%$ CI for the average rate estimate (equation 3.17) it is possible for the lower confidence limit to be negative. For modest sample sizes, one should use confidence intervals based on the natural logarithm of rate

$$\overline{\lambda}_1 \times \exp\left\{\pm z_{1-\alpha/2}\left(\sum_i e_i\right)^{-1/2}\right\}, \tag{3.18}$$

where $z_{1-\alpha/2}$ is the $100(1-\alpha)\%$th quantile of the standard normal distribution [52].

3.2.4 Probabilities of access

Definition

In health services research, where the interest lies in describing how quickly patients receive services, the primary tool for analysis is the access function, which shows the proportion of patients with waiting time T less than some stated value t and which thereby estimates the probability of undergoing surgery within a certain time t:

$$F(t) = \Pr(T < t). \tag{3.19}$$

In prospective studies, waiting times are analyzed as observations beginning at the time of registration, wait-list week 0, and followed up to removal, the last week on the list. Time to removal without surgery is then considered a censored observation, assuming that the actual wait would be larger otherwise [103].

Estimation

The cumulative probability of undergoing surgery within a certain time t, is commonly estimated using the complement of the product-limit method developed by Kaplan and Meier [17, 66]:

$$\hat{F}(t) = 1 - \prod_{\{i|t_i \leq t\}} \left(1 - \frac{e_i}{n_{i-1}}\right), \ t \geq t_1 . \tag{3.20}$$

Note that if no events have occurred by time t, then $\hat{F}(t) = 0$. In equation 3.20, $q_i = 1 - \frac{e_i}{n_{i-1}}$ is the conditional probability of not undergoing surgery during week i, and the cumulative product of q_i for all i such that $t_i \leq t$ estimates the probability of not undergoing surgery by time t.

The variance of the estimator at time t is given by

$$\widehat{\text{Var}}(\hat{F}(t)) = \left(1 - \hat{F}(t)\right)^2 \times \sum_{\{i|t_i \leq t\}} \frac{e_i}{n_{i-1}(n_{i-1} - e_i)} ,$$

and the standard error of the estimator is given by $\left(\widehat{\text{Var}}(\hat{F}(t))\right)^{1/2}$ at time t [66].

Interpretation

The graph of the access function, or access curve, is an informative visual tool for monitoring hospital wait-list statistics and studying access to surgery [78]. Figure 3.1 presents an example of an access curve that summarizes the probabilities of undergoing elective vascular surgery at a tertiary care center [103]. The abscissa shows time (in weeks) spent on the wait list since registration for surgery, and the ordinate shows the probability of undergoing the operation for each consecutive wait-list week.

The access curve, which is a nondecreasing function of time, provides many insights about the distribution of waiting times. First, one can specify a waiting time and determine the corresponding probability of undergoing surgery by this time. From a patient's perspective, the access curve displayed in Figure 3.1 shows that, according to historical performance, the chance of undergoing surgery by 13 weeks is 3 in 4. From a hospital's perspective, the same figure shows that 75% of patients will have to wait less than 13 weeks.

Second, one can determine the number of weeks required for a specified proportion of patients to undergo the operation. Figure 3.1 shows that 50% of patients underwent surgery in 6 weeks, the median time for the distribution of waits.

Third, one can compare the time between being registered on a wait list and undergoing surgery for equal proportions of patients in different groups. In Part II, we compare waiting times for elective vascular surgery across priority groups (Figure 6.1). The access curves in that figure show that half of the patients in priority groups 1, 2, 3, and 4 underwent surgery in 2, 3, 7, and 11 weeks, respectively.

Finally, one can compare access curves for specified wait-list intervals across periods to assess how access to elective CABG has changed during the decade (Figure 6.5). Table 6.4 shows the number of weeks required for a specified proportion of patients to undergo the operation across registration periods. Higher access probabilities in one period will be interpreted as representing shorter waiting times relative to another period. The access curves show that time to surgery increased in the middle of the decade and decreased toward the end of the decade. The access curve also shows the proportion of patients undergoing surgery within target access times: 8% within 1 week for patients with priority 1, 17% within 2 weeks for patients with priority 2, 27% within 3 weeks for patients with priority 3, and 16% within 4 weeks for patients with priority 4 (Figure 6.1).

Remarks

When dealing with censored observations, the sample average is not an appropriate summary measure of waiting times. For censored observations, it is assumed that actual waiting time for surgery is longer than

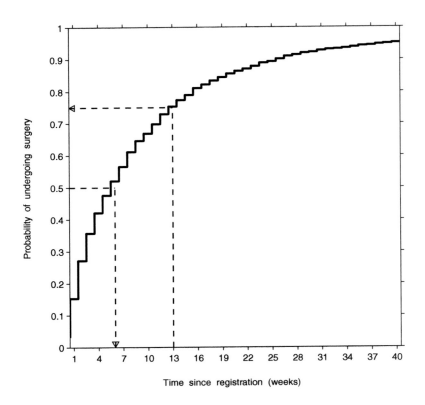

Fig. 3.1. Probability of undergoing elective vascular surgery within a certain waiting time, as estimated by the product-limit method

the observed follow-up time. Therefore, the sample average would result in an underestimate of the mean waiting time. An alternative to the mean waiting time is the median waiting time. The median waiting time to surgery is the length of time by which half of the patients undergo surgery. Unlike the mean, the median is not biased in the presence of censored observations. The median waiting time can be inferred from the access curve; it is the first week since registration when the probability of undergoing surgery exceeds 0.5 [66]. A related summary measure of interest is the median residual lifetime at time t defined as the period between time t and the time when one-half of the patients still remaining on the list at time t undergo surgery [66]. The median residual lifetime at time 0 is the median waiting time.

When there are competing events, the Kaplan-Meier method can also be used to estimate the probability of remaining on the list, $S(t)$, by certain times:

$$\hat{S}(t) = \prod_{\{i|t_i \leq t\}} \left(1 - \frac{e_i + r_i}{n_{i-1}}\right), \ t \geq t_1 . \tag{3.21}$$

Note that if no events have occurred by time t, then $\hat{S}(t) = 1$. In Part II, applications of the product-limit method to estimate the probabilities of remaining on the list are illustrated using waiting-time studies. For example, Figure 8.1 shows the estimated probabilities of remaining on the list for elective CABG by priority group.

When the product of the event-specific hazard, λ_m, and waiting time, t, is small, the cumulative hazard function is very close to the Kaplan-Meier estimator for the probability of event, since $1 - e^{-\lambda_m t} \approx \lambda_m t$. For instance, for patients waiting for elective CABG, the weekly probability of death before surgery is 0.0006, so the estimates of the cumulative hazard of death and the complement of the Kaplan-Meier curve for death are similar. In a competing-risks setting, caution should be exercised in using the Kaplan-Meier method for interpreting the estimated probabilities of a rare event, such as death on wait lists. In such cases, use of the Kaplan-Meier method is strongly discouraged. Instead, the cumulative incidence function, described in the next section, should be used.

In quantifying the risk of preoperative death among patients waiting for surgery, the Kaplan-Meier method is commonly used to estimate the cumulative probability of death by certain times after registration for the operation [58, 68, 94]. It has been established, however, that the Kaplan-Meier method is not appropriate for describing the probabilities of competing events, since its complement overestimates the event incidence [1]. This method produces valid probability estimates only in a hypothetical situation where all competing risks can be removed without altering the risk of death. Therefore, an alternative approach to summarizing wait-list data is to estimate the proportion of patients dying before surgery by a certain time and the proportion of patients dying by a certain time among those who have not received treatment by that time [73].

In the estimation of access curves, there is a difference in the information given by retrospective and prospective studies. Figure 3.2 shows the estimated probabilities of undergoing elective vascular surgery by a certain week since registration in the nonurgent group. Data for estimating these access curves were analyzed according to both a retrospective and a prospective design.

The difference between the estimates from the retrospective and prospective designs were measured by the one-sample log-rank test [41], described in section 3.3.4. Differences were statistically significant for the semiurgent (log-rank test = 3.7, df = 1, $p = 0.05$) and nonurgent (log-rank test = 49.1, df = 1, $p < 0.0001$), but not for the urgent group (log-rank test = 0.97, df = 1, $p = 0.33$). As expected, the retrospective analyses produced estimates of the probability of undergoing surgery that were biased upward. In these retrospective analyses, the average weekly admission rates were 46.4 per 100 patient-weeks (95% CI 41.4–51.4), 11.3 (95% CI 10.4–12.1), and 10.2 (95% CI 9.5–11.0) for the urgent, semiurgent and nonurgent groups, respectively. In contrast, in prospective analyses, the corresponding average weekly surgery rates were 43.5 per 100 patient-weeks (95% CI 38.8–48.2), 10.3 (95% CI 9.5–11.0), and 6.9 (95% CI 6.4–7.4).

Retrospective analyses also underestimated the median waiting times for surgery, which were 2 weeks (95% CI 1–2), 7 weeks (95% CI 7–8), and 7 weeks (95% CI 6–7) for the urgent, semiurgent, and nonurgent, respectively. In contrast, in prospective analyses, corresponding median wait times were 2 weeks (95% CI 1–2), 8 weeks (95% CI 7–8), and 8 weeks (95% CI 7–9).

3.2.5 Cumulative incidence functions

Definition

Methodologically, measuring the risk of death as a function of treatment delay among patients awaiting the treatment is similar to quantifying the risk of death during follow-up in a population exposed to competing

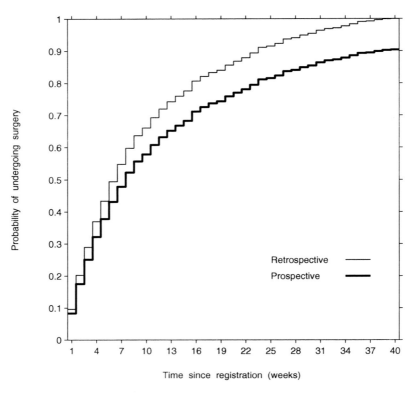

Fig. 3.2. Probability of undergoing surgery within a certain waiting time, as estimated by the product-limit method. Data for a single group of patients awaiting vascular surgery were analyzed according to both retrospective and prospective designs.

events [1]. One approach to summarizing competing-risks data is to estimate the proportion of patients dying by a certain time among those who have not received treatment by that time [73].

The cumulative incidence function (CIF) of event m,

$$F_m(t) = \Pr(T \le t, \delta = m) , \tag{3.22}$$

characterizes the time-dependent marginal probability that event m occurs at or before a certain waiting time in the presence of competing events. For instance, preoperative death or unplanned emergency surgery occurring before or during a certain week after registration on a wait list for surgery may be of interest.

The CIF of event m is calculated by the integration over time of the product of the event-specific hazard of event m and the probability of remaining on the list

$$F_m(t) = \int_0^t \lambda_m(u) S(u^-) \mathrm{d}u , \tag{3.23}$$

where $S(t^-) = \Pr(T > t^-)$ is the probability that a patient remains on the list beyond a time just before time t [21].

The CIF is also referred to as a subdistribution since it is not a proper distribution [91]. In a competing-risks setting the subdistribution of event m approaches the probability of event m as waiting time increases. In contrast, if there were no competing risks, the distribution would approach 1, a characteristic of a proper distribution.

Estimation

The CIF of an event and its standard errors can be estimated using nonparametric methods [90]. Kalbfleisch and Prentice suggested an estimator for the CIF of the primary event at discrete time t, $F_1(t)$, [59]:

$$\hat{F}_1(t) = \sum_{\{i|t_i \leq t\}} \frac{e_i}{n_{i-1}} \prod_{\{j|t_j \leq t_{i-1}\}} \left(1 - \frac{e_j + r_j}{n_{j-1}}\right). \tag{3.24}$$

The estimator

$$\hat{\lambda}_1(t_i) = \frac{e_i}{n_{i-1}} \tag{3.25}$$

represents the primary event hazard at time t_i, and

$$\hat{S}(t_{i-1}) = \prod_{\{j|t_j \leq t_{i-1}\}} \left(1 - \frac{e_j + r_j}{n_{j-1}}\right) \tag{3.26}$$

is the Kaplan-Meier estimator of the probability of remaining on the list beyond time t_{i-1}. The estimator in equation 3.24 is the maximum likelihood estimator [91].

Note that the probability of experiencing any event by time t is equal to the sum of all the cumulative incidences of the event at time t.

The standard error of the estimator for the CIF of the primary event is given by

$$\widehat{\text{SE}}(\hat{F}_1(t)) = \left(\widehat{\text{Var}}(\hat{F}_1(t))\right)^{1/2}. \tag{3.27}$$

Using a Taylor series approximation [43], the estimated variance of the estimator for the CIF of the primary event can be derived as follows,

$$\widehat{\text{Var}}(\hat{F}_1(t)) \approx \sum_{\{i|t_i \leq t\}} \left(\frac{n_{i-1} - e_i}{e_i n_{i-1}} + \sum_{\{j|t_j < t_i\}} \frac{e_j + r_j}{n_{j-1}(n_{j-1} - e_j - r_j)}\right) \times$$

$$\times \left(\frac{e_i}{n_{i-1}} \prod_{\{k|t_k \leq t_{i-1}\}} \left(1 - \frac{e_k + r_k}{n_{k-1}}\right)\right)^2 +$$

$$+ 2 \sum_{\{i|t_i < t\}} \left(-\frac{1}{n_{i-1}} + \sum_{\{j|t_j < t_i\}} \frac{e_j + r_j}{n_{j-1}(n_{j-1} - e_j - r_j)}\right) \frac{e_i}{n_{i-1}} \times$$

$$\times \prod_{\{k|t_k \leq t_{i-1}\}} \left(1 - \frac{e_k + r_k}{n_{k-1}}\right) \times \sum_{\{i'|t_{i'} \leq t\}} \frac{e_{i'}}{n_{i'-1}} \prod_{\{k|t_k \leq t_{i'-1}\}} \left(1 - \frac{e_k + r_k}{n_{k-1}}\right). \tag{3.28}$$

Pintilie has provided alternative estimators for the standard error of CIFs [91]. Nonparametric estimators for the CIF of the competing event are analogous.

Interpretation

We interpret the cumulative incidence of the primary event as the proportion of patients who experience the primary event before competing events, a value that increases with time on the wait list from which the patients can be removed because of any competing event. Since the CIF accounts for both the primary event rate and the waiting-time distribution, the impact of delay on the proportion of primary events can be evaluated.

In Part II, applications of the CIF are illustrated using waiting-time studies. For example, Figure 3.3 shows the estimated CIF of death among patients waiting for elective CABG. The ordinate shows the cumulative incidence of death on the wait list by a certain time and the abscissa shows week since registration on the wait list. From this figure, one can see that the percentage of patients who died on the wait lists by 52 weeks was 1.0%.

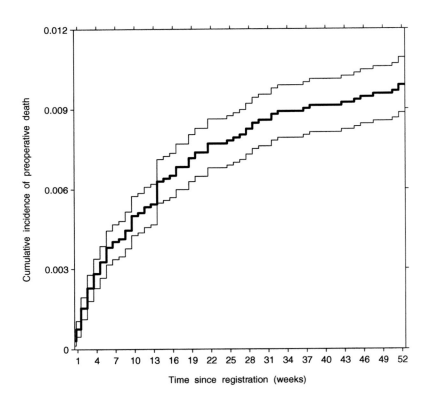

Fig. 3.3. Cumulative incidence of preoperative death during or before a certain week since registration for elective coronary artery bypass grafting, as estimated by the cumulative incidence function

Remarks

Gooley proposed an alternative form of the estimator for the CIF of the primary event:

$$\tilde{F}_1(t) = \sum_{\{i|t_i \leq t\}} e_i J(i)$$

where

$$J(i) = \begin{cases} \frac{1}{n_0}, & t \leq t_1 \\ J(i-1)\left(1 + \frac{c_{i-1}}{n_{i-1}}\right), & t > t_1 . \end{cases} \tag{3.29}$$

The relation between the two estimators is demonstrated by the following:

$$\hat{F}_1(t) = \sum_{\{i|t_i \leq t\}} \frac{e_i}{n_{i-1}} \prod_{\{j|t_j \leq t_{i-1}\}} \left(1 - \frac{e_j + r_j}{n_{j-1}}\right)$$

$$= \sum_{\{i|t_i \leq t\}} \frac{e_i}{n_{i-1}} \prod_{\{j|t_j \leq t_{i-1}\}} \left(\frac{n_{j-1} - (e_j + r_j)}{n_{j-1}}\right)$$

$$= \sum_{\{i|t_i \leq t\}} \frac{e_i}{n_{i-1}} \prod_{\{j|t_j \leq t_{i-1}\}} \left(\frac{(n_j + e_j + r_j + c_j) - (e_j + r_j)}{n_{j-1}}\right)$$

$$= \sum_{\{i|t_i \leq t\}} \frac{e_i}{n_{i-1}} \prod_{\{j|t_j \leq t_{i-1}\}} \left(\frac{n_j + c_j}{n_{j-1}}\right)$$

$$= \sum_{\{i|t_i \leq t\}} \frac{e_i}{n_{i-1}} \times \frac{(n_{i-1} + c_{i-1})}{n_0} \prod_{\{j|t_1 < t_j \leq t_{i-1}\}} \left(\frac{n_{j-1} + c_{j-1}}{n_{j-1}}\right)$$

$$= \sum_{\{i|t_i \leq t\}} \frac{e_i}{n_0} \prod_{\{j|t_1 < t_j \leq t_i\}} \left(1 + \frac{c_{j-1}}{n_{j-1}}\right)$$

$$= \tilde{F}_1(t) .$$

Although they yield the same estimate, the two formulations of the CIF estimator convey different messages. From the Kalbfleisch and Prentice estimator, $\hat{F}_1(t)$, it is apparent that the CIF estimator depends on the hazard of both the primary event and competing events. In addition, the CIF estimate at time t depends on the probability of remaining on the list. From the Gooley estimator, $\tilde{F}_1(t)$, it is apparent that the CIF of primary event estimate changes if and only if there is a primary event [45]. Note that if there were no censored observations, then the CIF would increase by $\frac{1}{n_0}$ for each observed primary event. However, if there are censored observations, their potential contribution to the primary event is distributed among patients who are still at risk.

CIFs are non-decreasing functions of waiting time that take values between 0 and 1. For the $100(1-\alpha)\%$ confidence interval for $\hat{F}_1(t)$ in equation 3.28, it is possible for the confidence limits to lie below 0 or exceed 1. An alternative $100(1-\alpha)\%$ confidence interval can be obtained by calculating the complementary log-log transformation of $\hat{F}_1(t)$. This confidence interval has the form [91]

$$\hat{F}(t)^{\exp(\pm\Gamma)} , \tag{3.30}$$

where

$$\Gamma = \frac{z_{1-\alpha/2}\sqrt{\widehat{\mathrm{Var}}(\hat{F}_1(t))}}{\hat{F}(t)\log(\hat{F}(t))} \; .$$

In quantifying the risk of adverse events on wait lists, the Kaplan-Meier method is commonly used to estimate the cumulative probability of an event by a certain time after registration for the operation [94, 58, 68]. It has been established, however, that the complement of the Kaplan-Meier estimator overestimates the incidence of the event in the competing risks setting [45, 91]. Because patients on wait lists are subject to competing events of surgery, death, or removal for other reasons, the method produces probability estimates that are valid only in a hypothetical situation when all competing risks are removed before the event without altering the risk of the adverse event of interest [43]. This implicitly assumes that time to surgery and time to the adverse event are independent. Without this assumption the Kaplan-Meier estimator is not valid and should not be used [1]. Furthermore, the independence of wait outcomes cannot be verified from data and may not be a realistic assumption, as low probability of the adverse event may indicate either low risk of this event or high surgery rate.

Pintilie proved that the cumulative incidence estimates are always less than or equal to the complement of the Kaplan-Meier curve to one $(1-\mathrm{KM})$ for all time points [91]. Figure 3.4 shows the estimated probabilities of preoperative death occurring during or before a certain week after registration for CABG, derived with (CIF) and without $(1-\mathrm{KM})$ adjustment for the incidence of all competing events. As expected, the two methods produced different estimates, with the CIF curve being lower than the $1-\mathrm{KM}$ curve. By 52 weeks on the list, the CIF curve reached the proportion of 0.009 and the $1-\mathrm{KM}$ curve reached 0.037.

Other investigators have reported the incidence of preoperative death per time unit of waiting for CABG [15, 80, 95, 94, 68, 33, 101]. Although accurately describing the instantaneous hazard, these death rates cannot be converted into the probabilities of death without the unrealistic and unverifiable assumption that time to surgery and time to death are independent [45]. Plomp et al. have reported on the variation in time to death among those who died before surgery [92], but the proportion of CABG candidates dying over follow-up could not be derived from their figures.

Appropriate statistical methods include the CIF, described in this section, and conditional probability function (CPF), described in the next section, which can be estimated without the independence assumption for competing events. CIF and CPF have been consistently suggested for summarizing results of time-to-event analysis with multiple competing end points [21, 24, 13]. Pepe argued that CIF is a more accurate and comprehensive summary of the risk of death in competing-risks settings than death rates or cumulative hazards, as the latter cannot be converted into death probabilities [90]. An alternative approach to summarizing competing-risks data is to estimate the proportion of patients dying by a certain time among those who have not received treatment by that time.

Given that CIFs estimate marginal probabilities, if the marginal probability of one event is low, then the marginal probability of the other will be high. CIFs for all events should be interpreted simultaneously. [90].

3.2.6 Conditional probability functions

Definition

Another approach suggested as a method for summarizing multiple end points in the competing-risks setting is to estimate the conditional probability function (CPF) [89]. For a primary event the CPF characterizes the probability that a patient will experience the event conditional on not experiencing the competing event in

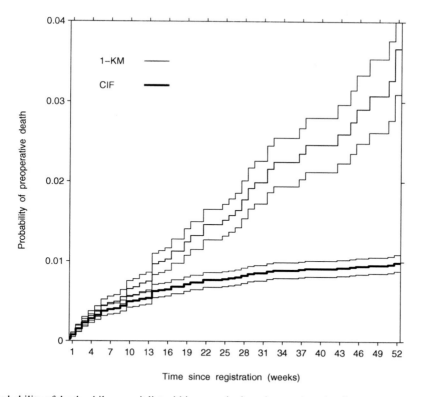

Fig. 3.4. Probability of death while on wait list within a certain time since registration for coronary artery bypass grafting, as estimated by the Kaplan-Meier method (1− KM) and the cumulative incidence function (CIF) (and standard errors)

relation to exposure time [90]. Let F_1 be the CIF of the primary event and F_2 be the CIF of the competing event. The CPF of the primary event, $CP_1(t)$, as a function of t is defined as

$$CP_1(t) = \frac{F_1(t)}{1 - F_2(t)} . \tag{3.31}$$

Estimation

To estimate CPF, one should first estimate separately the cumulative incidence of the primary event and the cumulative incidence of the competing event over time, while treating wait-list removals, other than those resulting from the primary event of interest and the competing event, as censored observations. The CPF of the primary event is then calculated by dividing the cumulative incidence of the primary event by the complement of cumulative incidence of the competing event [73]

$$\widehat{CP}_1(t) = \frac{\hat{F}_1(t)}{1 - \hat{F}_2(t)} . \tag{3.32}$$

In equation 3.32, the estimated CIF of the primary event is

$$\hat{F}_1 = \sum_{\{i|t_i \leq t\}} \frac{e_i}{n_{i-1}} \prod_{\{j|t_j \leq t_{i-1}\}} \left(1 - \frac{e_j + r_j}{n_{j-1}}\right) , \tag{3.33}$$

and the estimated CIF of the competing event is

$$\hat{F}_2 = \sum_{\{i|t_i \leq t\}} \frac{r_i}{n_{i-1}} \prod_{\{j|t_j \leq t_{i-1}\}} \left(1 - \frac{e_j + r_j}{n_{j-1}}\right) . \tag{3.34}$$

Notice that the competing event may occur at times different from the primary event.

Pepe [90] showed that $\sqrt{n}\{\widehat{CP}_1(t) - CP_1(t)\} \sim N(0, \sigma^2(t))$, where a consistent variance estimator for $\sigma^2(t)$ is given by

$$\begin{aligned}
\hat{\sigma}^2(t) &= \frac{[\hat{S}(t)]^2}{[1 - \hat{F}_2(t)]^4} \int_0^t \frac{[1 - \hat{F}_2(t_u)]^2 dN_1(u) + [\hat{F}_1(t_u)]^2 dN_2(u)}{n_{u-1}[n_{u-1} - 1]/n_0} \\
&\approx \frac{[\hat{S}(t)]^2}{[1 - \hat{F}_2(t)]^4} \sum_{\{i|t_i \leq t\}} \frac{[1 - \hat{F}_2(t_i)]^2 e_i + [\hat{F}_1(t_i)]^2 r_i}{n_{i-1}[n_{i-1} - 1]/n_0} .
\end{aligned} \tag{3.35}$$

Here, $N_1(k)$ and $N_2(k)$ are the number of primary events and competing events that have occurred up to and including time t_k, respectively.

Therefore, an approximate $100(1 - \alpha)\%$ confidence interval for $CP_1(t)$ is

$$\widehat{CP}_1(t) \pm z_{\alpha/2} \frac{\hat{\sigma}(t)}{\sqrt{n_0}} , \tag{3.36}$$

where $z_{\alpha/2}$ is the $100(1 - \alpha/2)$th quantile of the standard normal distribution.

Interpretation

The CPF of the primary event is interpreted as the cumulative incidence of the primary event by a certain wait-list week among patients not experiencing the competing event by that time. The risk of an adverse event as a function of treatment delay is described by the probability that a patient experiences the adverse event, conditional on not receiving surgery by a certain time after registration on a wait list.

In Part II, applications of CPF are illustrated using waiting-time studies. For example, Figure 8.10 shows the estimated conditional probability of preoperative death by time since registration for elective CABG. The ordinate shows the conditional probability of death by a certain time, and the abscissa shows time since registration on the wait list. Among patients who had not undergone CABG by 52 weeks, the probabilities of death were 0.14 and 0.08 in the semiurgent and nonurgent groups, respectively.

Remarks

CPFs may range from 0 to 1. For the $100(1 - \alpha)\%$ confidence interval for $\widehat{CP}_1(t)$ in equation 3.36, it is possible for the confidence limits to lie below 0 or exceed 1. An alternative $100(1 - \alpha)\%$ confidence interval is given by the complementary log-log transformation of $\widehat{CP}_1(t)$. This confidence interval has the form [91]

$$\widehat{CP}_1(t)^{\exp(\pm\Gamma)},\tag{3.37}$$

where

$$\Gamma = \frac{z_{1-\alpha/2}\sqrt{\widehat{\mathrm{Var}}(\widehat{CP}_1(t))}}{\hat{F}(t)\log(\widehat{CP}_1(t))}.$$

3.3 Methods of comparison

3.3.1 Notation

In this section, we use notation defined in section 3.2.1. Although we consider only two types of events, the primary event and the competing event, this does not restrict generality since events other than the primary event may be combined into a single competing risk [91].

3.3.2 Comparison of proportions and odds

In section 3.2.2 we introduced proportions and odds as summary measures for a binary outcome where the event occurred or did not occur, for example, the patient underwent surgery or did not undergo surgery after registration on a wait list. To determine and quantify differences in proportions or odds between groups, measures of comparison are required. In this section, we describe methods for comparing proportions and odds between groups.

Pearson's test of association

Pearson's test is used to test for an association between binary outcomes and group membership. The null hypothesis states that there is no association, whereas the alternative hypothesis states that there is an association. The general form for the Pearson's test statistic is based upon differences between observed and expected counts [29]:

$$S^2 = \sum_i \sum_j \frac{(O_{ij} - E_{ij})^2}{E_{ij}},\tag{3.38}$$

where O_{ij} is the observed count and E_{ij} is the expected count in row i and column j of the contingency table, in which i indexes group ($i = 1, \ldots, g$), and j indexes outcome ($j \in \{\text{event, no event}\}$). Expected counts, E_{ij}, are derived under the assumption of the null hypothesis that the probability of an event across the groups are equal. For example, the expected number of events in group 1 is the product of the number of patients in group 1 and the overall observed proportion of events in all groups.

Under the null hypothesis, the test statistic in equation 3.38 has a chi-square distribution with $g - 1$ degrees of freedom [29]. A value of the test statistic greater than the $100(1 - \alpha)$th percentile of the chi-square distribution with $g - 1$ degrees of freedom indicates that there is sufficient evidence to reject the null hypothesis at the α significance level. For example, with two groups at the 0.05 significance level, the 95th percentile of a chi-square distribution with 1 degree of freedom is 3.84. The probability of observing a value greater than the test statistic given the null hypothesis is called the p-value. By convention, small p-values are interpreted as evidence against the null hypothesis. The p-value is computed from the chi-square distribution with $g - 1$ degrees of freedom.

Odds ratios

In section 3.2.2 we introduced the concept of odds of an event. The odds ratio (OR) is the ratio of the odds for one group to the odds for another group:

$$OR = \frac{\text{odds for group } 1}{\text{odds for group } 2}. \tag{3.39}$$

The ORs are commonly used in health services research to quantify differences between two groups. If the OR is 1, then the odds of the event is the same in the two groups. If the OR is greater than 1, then the odds of the event is higher in group 1 than in group 2, whereas if the OR is less than 1, then the odds of the event is lower in group 1 than in group 2. The OR is estimated by the ratio of the estimated odds [55]:

$$\widehat{OR} = \frac{\hat{p}_1/(1 - \hat{p}_1)}{\hat{p}_2/(1 - \hat{p}_2)}, \tag{3.40}$$

where $\hat{p}_1$ and $\hat{p}_2$ are the estimated event proportions in groups 1 and 2, respectively. Group 2 is often called the reference group.

Determining if the odds of an event differs between two groups is equivalent to testing whether the OR differs from 1 or whether the logarithm of OR differs from 0. Statistical tests for differences in the odds between groups are based on the quantity $\beta = \log(OR)$ since it has an approximately normal distribution [55, 52]. The Wald test statistic is then

$$W = \frac{\hat{\beta}}{SE(\hat{\beta})}, \tag{3.41}$$

where $\hat{\beta}$ is $\log(\widehat{OR})$, $SE(\hat{\beta})$ is the standard error of $\hat{\beta}$, and W^2 has a chi-square distribution with 1 degree of freedom [55]. Estimators for $SE(\hat{\beta})$ may be found in Hosmer and Lemeshow [55] or Holford [52]. A W^2 value greater than the $100(1 - \alpha)$th percentile of the chi-square distribution with 1 degree of freedom indicates that there is sufficient evidence to reject the null hypothesis at the α significance level. At the 0.05 significance level, the 95th percentile of a chi-square distribution with 1 degree of freedom is 3.84.

A $100(1 - \alpha)\%$ CI for $\widehat{OR}$ is given by

$$\exp\{\hat{\beta} \pm z_{1-\alpha/2} \times SE(\hat{\beta})\}, \tag{3.42}$$

where $z_{1-\alpha/2}$ is the $100(1 - \alpha/2)$th quantile of the standard normal distribution.

Remarks

Pearson's test of association is an attractive approach for comparing proportions since it can be computed by essentially all statistical programs and is easily extended to more than two groups. For a valid chi-square test, one should ensure that the expected counts must be greater than 5 [29]. In the case of a binary outcome and two groups, the chi-square test is based on the normal approximate to the binomial distribution, therefore, Yate's correction should be applied, which involves subtracting 0.5 from the absolute value of the difference between observed and expected counts.

ORs allow not only testing of hypotheses but also quantification of the relative difference in outcomes. There is a relation between hypothesis tests at the α significance level and $100(1-\alpha)\%$ confidence intervals. If the null hypothesis that OR $= 1$ is rejected at the α level, then the $100(1 - \alpha)\%$ confidence interval for the OR will not contain 1. Conversely, if the null hypothesis is not rejected, then the confidence interval for the OR will contain 1. We emphasize that confidence intervals are more informative than simply reporting a p-value.

3.3.3 Comparison of hazard and event rates

Hazard ratios

In section 3.2.3, we defined the hazard as the instantaneous probability of an event at time t, conditional on remaining at risk of the event by that time (for example, conditional on the patient remaining on the wait list until that time). Recall that the term "hazard" is used to refer to a continuous-time setting. The hazard ratio (HR) is the ratio of the hazard for one group to the hazard for another group

$$\text{HR} = \frac{\text{hazard for group 1}}{\text{hazard for group 2}} . \tag{3.43}$$

The HR quantifies the relative hazard of an event in two groups and, therefore, comparing the HR to 1 is used to describe differences between groups. If the HR is 1, then the hazard of the event is the same in the two groups. If the HR is greater than 1, then the hazard of the event is higher in group 1 than in group 2, whereas if the HR is less than 1, then the hazard of the event is lower in group 1 than in group 2.

The hazard function of continuous time is a theoretical construct and cannot be estimated directly from data. As described in section 3.4.3, Cox regression can be used to model the hazard of an event and to obtain the HRs and their corresponding CIs for making comparisons between groups.

Rate ratios

In section 3.2.3, we introduced the concept of event rate. The rate ratio (RR) is the ratio of the event rate for one group to the rate for another group:

$$\text{RR} = \frac{\text{event rate for group 1}}{\text{event rate for group 2}} . \tag{3.44}$$

The RR measures relative differences in the rate of an event between two groups. If the RR is 1, then the event-specific rate is the same in the two groups. If the RR is greater than 1, then the rate is higher in group 1 than in group 2, whereas if the RR is less than 1, then the rate is lower in group 1 than in group 2. Therefore, comparing rates in two groups is equivalent to comparing the RR to 1. The RR is estimated by the ratio of the estimated rates:

$$\widehat{\text{RR}} = \frac{E_1/T_1}{E_2/T_2}, \tag{3.45}$$

where E_1, E_2 are the total count of events and T_1, T_2 are the total times at risk in groups 1 and 2, respectively. As described in section 3.4.4, Poisson regression can be used to obtain the RRs and their corresponding CIs for comparing multiple groups. In addition, it is possible to test the hypothesis that the rates in two groups are different.

Odds ratios for discrete times

In waiting-time studies, researchers are often interested in events occurring over time, where time is (or considered) discrete. In section 3.2.3, we introduced the conditional probability of an event as a measure of discrete-time hazard. Recall that the conditional probability is estimated by a proportion, where the numerator is the number of events in a given period and the denominator is the number of patients at risk (see equation 3.2). In this context, the OR measures the relative conditional odds of an event of interest in two groups at time t among those who are still at risk by that time. The OR for discrete times t is the ratio of the conditional odds of the event for one group to the conditional odds for another group:

$$OR_t = \frac{\text{conditional odds of event for group 1}}{\text{conditional odds of event for group 2}} . \tag{3.46}$$

For events occurring on wait lists, the OR for week t since registration is estimated by the ratio of the estimated conditional odds:

$$\widehat{OR}_t = \frac{\hat{p}_{1t}/(1 - \hat{p}_{1t})}{\hat{p}_{2t}/(1 - \hat{p}_{2t})} , \tag{3.47}$$

where $\hat{p}_{gt}$ is the estimated event proportion in week t among patients who were still remaining on the list until that week in group $g = 1, 2$.

If the difference between two groups is assumed to be constant over consecutive follow-up periods, a common OR can be estimated using discrete-time survival regressions in which the log odds for the reference groups are modeled for each period of follow-up (see section 3.4.5).

3.3.4 Comparison of probabilities of access

Log-rank test

In section 3.2.4, we introduced the concept of access probabilities, which represent the probabilities of undergoing surgery within certain times from registration. These cumulative probabilities can be estimated using the Kaplan-Meier method. Suppose we are interested in comparing the chances of undergoing surgery within a certain time across groups, for instance, to determine if classifying patients into urgency groups makes a difference in times to surgery.

By using the log-rank test, access to surgery can be compared across patient groups [18, 66]. The log-rank test is a nonparametric test based on the difference between the observed and expected number of procedures in each group [66]. Using the notation from section 3.3.1, the contribution to the test statistic from group g is

$$\sum_{j=1}^{E} \left(e_{gj} - \frac{e_j}{n_{j-1}} \times n_{g,j-1} \right) , \tag{3.48}$$

where e_{gj} is the observed number of procedures (the primary event) in group g at time t_j, and $n_{g,j-1}$ is the number of patients in group g who are still waiting beyond time t_{j-1}.

The null hypothesis states that the access curves across groups are the same. Under the null hypothesis, the log-rank test statistic has a chi-square distribution with degrees of freedom equal to one fewer than the number of groups being compared [59]. At the 0.05 significance level, a p-value less than 0.05 indicates that there is sufficient evidence to support the hypothesis that the access curves are different. For further details, see Klein and Moeschberger [66].

Wilcoxon test

The nonparametric Wilcoxon test can be used to compare access to surgery across patient groups. The Wilcoxon test is based on a weighted difference between the observed and expected numbers of procedures in each group [66]. Using notation from section 3.3.1, the contribution to the test statistic from group g is

$$\sum_{j=1}^{E} n_{j-1} \left(e_{gj} - \frac{e_j}{n_{j-1}} \times n_{g,j-1} \right), \tag{3.49}$$

where e_{gj} is the observed number of procedures (the primary event) in group g and time t_j, and $n_{g,j-1}$ is the number of patients in group g, who are still waiting beyond time t_{j-1}. Note that the weight is equal to n_{j-1} which is the total number of patients who are still waiting beyond time t_{j-1}.

The null hypothesis states that the access curves across groups are the same. Under the null hypothesis, the Wilcoxon test statistic has a chi-square distribution with degrees of freedom equal to one fewer than the number of groups being compared [59]. At the 0.05 significance level, a p-value less than 0.05 indicates that there is sufficient evidence to support the hypothesis that the access curves are different. For further details, see Klein and Moeschberger [66].

Remarks

The Wilcoxon test differs from the log-rank test since it is a weighted sum of differences between the observed and expected numbers of events. This weight is equal to the number of patients remaining on the list at a certain time. Since these weights are greater for early time points, the Wilcoxon test is more sensitive to differences at earlier times than the log-rank test [3]. The log-rank test and the Wilcoxon test do not do well in detecting differences when the access curves cross [3].

The log-rank test is suitable for comparing two or more groups. In some cases, it may be of interest to compare one group with a standard population. In this case, comparisons can be made using the one-sample log-rank test [41], which is based on the difference between the total observed number of events, O, and total expected number of events, E. The total expected number of events is equal to the sum of the cumulative event rate (equation 3.9) at the time of last follow-up for each patient. The one-sample log-rank statistic is

$$\frac{(O - E)^2}{E}. \tag{3.50}$$

The null hypothesis states that the access curve in the group of interest is the same as that of the standard population. Under the null hypothesis, the one-sample log-rank statistic has a chi-square distribution with one degree of freedom.

The cumulative probability of removal for any reason within a certain time after registration can also be estimated using the product–limit method [17]. By using the log-rank test or the Wilcoxon test, time to removal is compared across groups [18].

3.3.5 Comparison of cumulative incidence functions

In section 3.2.5, we introduced the CIF as an appropriate measure for summarizing the risk of an event in a wait-list setting. Suppose we want to compare the proportions of patients experiencing an adverse event, such as preoperative death, by a certain time between groups. In this section, we discuss methods for comparing CIFs.

Two-sample test

Using Gray's two-sample test, it is possible to compare CIFs between study groups [47]. This method tests the hypothesis of equality of CIFs across groups by comparing weighted averages of the hazards of the subdistributions. An open-source R code for the estimation and comparison of CIFs has been developed by Gray [46]. For further details, see Gray [47] and Pintilie [91].

Nonparametric two-sample test

Using a nonparametric, two-sample test, CIFs can be compared across groups by the methods developed by Pepe [90]. The test statistic is a cumulative weighted differences between CIFs. For discrete times, the test statistic is

$$\Delta = \left(\frac{n^I n^{II}}{n^I + n^{II}} \right)^{1/2} \sum_{\{i|t_i>0\}} \hat{W}(t_i)(\hat{F}_1^I(t_i) - \hat{F}_1^{II}(t_i))(t_i - t_{i-1}) \,,$$

where n^g is the number of patients in group g, $\hat{F}_1^g(t)$ is the estimated CIF of the primary event for group g at time t, and the weight function, $\hat{W}(t_i)$, is calculated from data as follows

$$\hat{W}(t_i) = \hat{C}^I(t_i)\hat{C}^{II}(t_i) \left(\frac{n^I}{n^I + n^{II}}\hat{C}^I(t_i) + \frac{n^{II}}{n^I + n^{II}}\hat{C}^{II}(t_i) \right)^{-1} \,, \tag{3.51}$$

where $\hat{C}^g(t)$ is the left-continuous estimator of the censoring distribution function in group g at time t, and $g = I, II$. This choice of the weight function reduces the impact of differences at later time points, when the number of patients still on the list is small.

Pepe showed that the asymptotic distribution of Δ is normal, with a mean of zero. The variance estimator

$$\frac{n^{II}}{n^I + n^{II}}\hat{\sigma}_I^2 + \frac{n^I}{n^I + n^{II}}\hat{\sigma}_{II}^2 \tag{3.52}$$

converges in probability to the true variance. Here (suppressing group subscripts and superscripts),

$$\hat{\sigma}_i^2 = n \sum_{\{i|t_i>0\}} \frac{1}{n_{i-1}(n_{i-1}-1)} \left\{ \left[\sum_{\{j|t_j\geq t_i\}} \hat{W}(t_j)\{1-\hat{F}_1(t_j)-\hat{F}_2(t_i)\} \right]^2 e_i + \left[\sum_{\{j|t_j\geq t_i\}} \hat{W}(t_j)\hat{F}_1(t_j) \right]^2 r_i \right\} \,,$$

where $n = n^I + n^{II}$.

Remarks

Gray's two-sample test can be used to compare CIFs across two or more groups. Lunn extended Pepe's two-sample test to compare CIFs across multiple groups [75].

Recall that the CIF depends on both the event-specific rate and the probability of remaining on the list. This observation may help in the interpretation of differences between CIFs. For example, if the primary event of interest is preoperative death and if the CIF for preoperative death differs between two groups but the death rates are the same, then it is the probabilities of remaining on the list that contribute to the difference. Alternatively, if the primary event of interest is unplanned emergency surgery and the rate of emergency surgery is higher in one of the groups while the CIFs are similar, then it is the lower probabilities of remaining on the list that contribute to the similarity.

3.3.6 Comparison of conditional probability functions

In section 3.2.6, we introduced the CPF as an appropriate measure for summarizing the risk of an event in a competing-risks setting. Suppose we would like to compare proportions of patients experiencing an adverse event by a certain time on the wait list among those who had not undergone surgery by that time. In this section, we present methods for comparing conditional probabilities over time.

Nonparametric two-sample test

Using a nonparametric, two-sample test, CPFs are compared between the study groups by methods developed by Pepe [90]. Suppose there are two competing events. Let F_1 be the CIF for event 1 and F_2 be the CIF for event 2. Let the CPF for event 1, $CP_1(t)$, be defined as follows:

$$CP_1(t) = \frac{\Pr(\text{event 1 by time } t)}{1 - \Pr(\text{event 2 by time } t)}$$
$$= \frac{F_1(t)}{1 - F_2(t)} .$$

A statistic developed by Pepe can be used to test the hypothesis that the CPF of event 1 is greater in group I than in group II [90]. The statistic is a cumulative weighted difference between CPFs. For discrete time, this test statistic is

$$\Delta = \left(\frac{n^I n^{II}}{n^I + n^{II}} \right)^{1/2} \sum_{\{i|t_i>0\}} \hat{W}(t_i)(\widehat{CP}_1^I(t_i) - \widehat{CP}_1^{II}(t_i))(t_i - t_{i-1}) , \tag{3.53}$$

where $\widehat{CP}_1^g(t)$ denotes the estimated CPF for group g at time t, n^g is the number of patients in group g, and the weight function, $\hat{W}(t_i)$, is as follows

$$\hat{W}(t_i) = \hat{C}^I(t_i)\hat{C}^{II}(t_i) \left(\frac{n^I}{n^I + n^{II}}\hat{C}^I(t_i) + \frac{n^{II}}{n^I + n^{II}}\hat{C}^{II}(t_i) \right)^{-1} , \tag{3.54}$$

where $\hat{C}^g(t)$ is the left-continuous estimator of the censoring distribution function in group g at time t, and $g = I, II$. This choice of the weight function reduces the impact of differences at later time points, when the number of patients still on the list is small.

Under the null hypothesis that the CPFs in both groups are equal, Pepe showed that the asymptotic distribution of Δ is normal, with a mean of zero and variance $\rho^{II}\sigma_I^2 + \rho^I\sigma_{II}^2$, where $\rho^g = \lim_{n\to\infty} \frac{n^g}{n^I+n^{II}}$.

The variance estimator,

$$\frac{n^{II}}{n^I + n^{II}}\hat{\sigma}_I^2 + \frac{n^I}{n^I + n^{II}}\hat{\sigma}_{II}^2 , \tag{3.55}$$

converges in probability to the true variance. Here (suppressing group subscripts and superscripts),

$$\hat{\sigma}^2 = n \sum_{\{i|t_i>0\}} \left\{ \left[\sum_{\{j|t_j\geq t_i\}} \frac{\hat{W}(t_j)\hat{S}(t_j)(t_j - t_{j-1})}{[1 - \hat{F}_2(t_j)]^2} \right]^2 \left[\frac{[1 - \hat{F}_2(t_i)]^2 e_i + [\hat{F}_1(t_i)]^2 r_i}{n_{i-1}(n_{i-1} - 1)} \right] \right\} , \tag{3.56}$$

where $n = n^I + n^{II}$.

Remarks

Pepe's nonparametric test for comparing conditional probabilities over time can be extended to more than two groups [75, 91].

3.4 Regression models

In health services research, regression models are used to quantify the effect of one variable after adjustment for other variables.

3.4.1 Notation

Suppose there is a synthetic cohort of n patients who registered on the wait lists for surgery during some calendar period. Let x_{ij} be the value of covariate j for patient i, where $j = 1, \ldots, m$. Let t_i be the waiting time and δ_i be the indicator for a noncensored event for patient i. Without loss of generality, it is assumed that time is measured in calendar weeks. The notation for the response variable is defined for each model below.

3.4.2 Logistic regression

In section 3.2.2, we defined the proportion and described its relation to the odds of an event. The odds ratio (OR) as a measure of comparison between two groups was described in section 3.3.2. In this section, we introduce a regression model to quantify the effect of a study variable with adjustment for other factors using ORs.

Logistic regression models the relation between a binary outcome and one or more explanatory variables [55]. Examples of binary outcomes include whether or not the patient received surgery within the target access time, and whether the patient died while on the wait list. Explanatory variables of interest might be priority group or wait-list size. Logistic regression helps in addressing questions such as "How much more likely is it that a patient with urgent status will die on the wait list than a patient with nonurgent status?"

Model

Let y_i be the value of a binary outcome variable, 1 or 0, for patient i, with a value of 1 indicating that the event of interest occurred and a value of 0 indicating that the event did not occur. The adjusted effect of a factor on the proportion of patients experiencing the event can be estimated by means of logistic regression that models the log odds of the probability p_i that patient i experiences the event, or the probability that y_i equals 1, as a linear function of covariates

$$\log\left(\frac{p_i}{1 - p_i}\right) = \alpha + \beta_1 x_{i1} + \ldots + \beta_m x_{im} , \tag{3.57}$$

where $\alpha, \beta_1, \ldots, \beta_m$ are the model parameters; β_j is a regression coefficient associated with covariate j and the intercept α is the log odds in a reference group. Note that this model implies that the probability of the event depends on the explanatory variables [55]. The expression on the left-hand side of equation 3.57 is referred to as the logit of p_i.

The binary outcome variable is assumed to have a binomial distribution, therefore maximum likelihood techniques can be used to estimate the model parameters. The method involves finding a set of parameters that maximize the probability of observing the given data, which, when considered a function of the model parameters, is called the likelihood function. The likelihood function for the logistic regression model is

$$L(\alpha, \beta_1, \ldots, \beta_m) = \prod_{i=1}^{n} p_i^{y_i} (1 - p_i)^{1-y_i} \,, \tag{3.58}$$

where $p_i = (1 + \exp\{-(\alpha + \beta_1 x_{i1} + \ldots + \beta_m x_{im})\})^{-1}$ [4]. This approach assumes that the patients are independent of each other. Maximum likelihood estimates of these parameters can be obtained by using SAS PROC LOGISTIC or PROC GENMOD.

Once the model is estimated, one of the first questions to be addressed is "Does the model with covariates explain the outcome better than a model with no covariates at all?" The likelihood ratio test can be used to assess goodness of fit, by testing the hypothesis that at least one of the regression coefficients is different from 0. The test statistic compares the observed and predicted values via the likelihood function [55]:

$$\text{LRT} = -2\log\left(\frac{\text{likelihood of model with intercept only}}{\text{likelihood of fitted model}}\right). \tag{3.59}$$

Under the global null hypothesis, in which all regression coefficients are 0, the test statistic follows a chi-square distribution with degrees of freedom equal to m. If the null hypothesis is rejected, it can be concluded that at least one of the covariates is associated with the outcome.

Once it has been determined that the model with covariates is better than no model at all, it is possible to evaluate specifically which covariates are associated with the outcome. The Wald test can be used to test the hypothesis that the model parameter is different from 0. The Wald test statistic is

$$W = \frac{\hat{\beta}_j}{\text{SE}(\hat{\beta}_j)} \,, \tag{3.60}$$

where $\hat{\beta}_j$ is the parameter estimate for the jth explanatory variable and $\text{SE}(\hat{\beta}_j)$ is the standard error of $\hat{\beta}_j$. Under the null hypothesis that $\beta_j = 0$, W^2 has a chi-square distribution with 1 degree of freedom. Along with the point estimates, statistical software provides their standard errors.

A $100(1 - \alpha)\%$ confidence interval for β_j is given by

$$\hat{\beta}_j \pm z_{1-\alpha/2} \times \text{SE}(\hat{\beta}_j) \,, \tag{3.61}$$

where $z_{1-\alpha/2}$ is the $100(1 - \alpha/2)$th quantile of the standard normal distribution.

Interpretation

The regression coefficients in the logistic model (equation 3.57) quantify association between the explanatory variables and the log odds of the event of interest. The regression estimates themselves, $\hat{\beta}_j$, may be difficult to interpret. However, these estimates are related to a more familiar measure of comparison, namely OR, described in section 3.3.2. For a binary explanatory variable, x_j, for which one category is coded as 1 and the reference category is coded as 0, the exponential of the estimate $\hat{\beta}_j$

$$\widehat{\text{OR}} = \exp\{\hat{\beta}_j\} \,, \tag{3.62}$$

produces the OR that compares the odds of the event in patients with $x_j = 1$ to the odds of the event in patients with $x_j = 0$. For example, when the event is surgery and the variable x_j represents sex with a value of 1 for a woman and a value of 0 for a man, the OR less than 1 indicates lower odds of undergoing surgery in women relative to men. In general, if OR is 1, there is no difference in the odds of the event. If OR is greater than 1, the odds of the event are greater, and if OR is less than 1, the odds are lower. An approximate $100(1 - \alpha)\%$ CI for this OR is given by

$$\exp\left\{\hat{\beta}_j \pm z_{1-\alpha/2} \times \text{SE}(\hat{\beta}_j)\right\}. \tag{3.63}$$

Note that this CI needs not be symmetric around the point estimate $\exp\{\hat{\beta}_j\}$.

For a continuous variable, using the maximum likelihood estimate $\hat{\beta}_j$, the effect of an increase in value by δ units is estimated by

$$\widehat{\text{OR}} = \exp\left\{\hat{\beta}_j \times \delta\right\}, \tag{3.64}$$

and its approximate $100(1 - \alpha)\%$ CI is given by

$$\exp\left\{\hat{\beta}_j \times \delta \pm z_{1-\alpha/2} \times \delta \times \text{SE}(\hat{\beta}_j)\right\}, \tag{3.65}$$

which is not symmetric around the point estimate. This OR compares the odds of the event between groups of patients with values of the continuous variable that differ by δ units. Typically, δ is taken to be 1, such that the change in odds is for every unit increase of the continuous variable. For example, if the variable x_j represents age in years and $\delta = 1$, then $\exp\{\hat{\beta}_j \times 1\}$ represents the factor by which the odds changes for every year of increase in age.

Studies in health services research often report the quantity $100 \times |e^{\hat{\beta}_j} - 1|$ that estimates the percentage change in odds for a 1-unit increase in continuous covariate x_j [4]. For a binary covariate, $100 \times |e^{\hat{\beta}_j} - 1|$ similarly estimates the percentage change in odds in one group relative to the reference group.

Remarks

The motivation for using a logit transformation in logistic regression arises from the fact that the probability of an event can only range from 0 to 1. Directly modeling a probability using a linear regression model would be inappropriate, as estimates could lie below 0 or above 1, whereas modeling the logit of a probability restricts probability estimates to lie between 0 and 1. For a complete discussion of logistic regression, refer to Hosmer and Lemeshow [55]. In Part II, we use logistic regression in the analysis of registration outcomes for patients on the wait list. In Chapter 8, we compare the odds of preoperative death at 52 weeks in the semiurgent and nonurgent groups. The odds of death at 52 weeks were about 1.6 times greater in the nonurgent group than in the semiurgent group (OR = 1.6, 95% CI 1.0–2.6).

When interpreting ORs for continuous variables, a meaningful unit of change should be used. For example, if the number of direct admissions is an explanatory variable of interest, it may be more meaningful to consider the OR associated with an increase in the mean weekly number of direct admissions than interpret the OR associated with an increase of one direct admission.

Note that $\log(\text{OR}) = \log(e^\beta) = \beta$ and $\log(1) = 0$; therefore, testing the hypothesis that OR is different from 1 is equivalent to testing the hypothesis that β is different from 0. There is a relation between CIs and hypothesis tests. If the null hypothesis that OR is 1 is rejected at the α significance level, then the $100(1 - \alpha)\%$ CI for the OR will not contain 1. Conversely, if the null hypothesis is not rejected, then the CI for the OR will contain 1.

3.4.3 Cox regression

In section 3.2.3, we introduced the concept of hazard and later in section 3.3.3 the hazard ratio (HR) was defined as a measure of comparison between two groups. In this section we discuss the use of proportional hazards models for obtaining adjusted HRs associated with study variables. Cox proportional hazards models are widely used in a variety of survival analysis applications to explore association between the hazard of an event and one or more explanatory variables. For example, suppose the primary event of interest is death. It may be of interest to study how treating patients with surgery affects their risk of death. In this scenario, the Cox model is used to estimate the expected percentage change in the hazard of death in treated relative to untreated patients. Cox regression models may be applied to both continuous and discrete time data. Here, we describe the model for continuous time, which we use for the analysis of times to death.

Model

The adjusted HR can be obtained from the Cox regression that models the hazard of an event for patient i at time t as the product of the baseline hazard, $\lambda_0(t)$, and an exponentiated linear function of covariates

$$\lambda_i(t) = \lambda_0(t) \exp\{\beta_1 x_{i1} + \cdots + \beta_m x_{im}\}, \tag{3.66}$$

where $\beta_1, \ldots, \beta_m$ are regression coefficients associated with the covariates and the baseline hazard function $\lambda_0(t)$ can be thought of as the hazard for a reference group [31]. One appealing feature of the model is its semiparametric nature; the form of the baseline hazard function does not have to be specified but needs to be restricted to a value greater than 0. Second, the covariates have a multiplicative effect on the hazard function. Third, this model is often referred to as a "proportional hazards" model since the ratio of two patients' hazards is assumed to be proportional over time.

Although for this model it does not have to be assumed that waiting times follow a specific distribution, the maximum likelihood method still can be used to estimate the model parameters. The partial likelihood function of the proportional hazards model with fixed covariates is

$$PL(\beta_1, \ldots, \beta_m) = \prod_{i=1}^{n} \left(\frac{e^{\beta_1 x_{i1} + \cdots + \beta_m x_{im}}}{\sum_{\{j|t_j \geq t_i\}} e^{\beta_1 x_{j1} + \ldots + \beta_m x_{jm}}} \right)^{\delta_i}, \tag{3.67}$$

which does not include the baseline hazard function $\lambda_0(t)$ [3]. In practice, statistical programs, such as SAS PROC PHREG, can be used to obtain parameter estimates.

The Wald test is used to test the hypothesis that a model parameter is different from 0. The Wald test statistic is the ratio of the parameter estimate to its standard error:

$$W = \frac{\hat{\beta}_j}{\mathrm{SE}(\hat{\beta}_j)}, \tag{3.68}$$

where $\hat{\beta}_j$ is the parameter estimate for the jth covariate and $\mathrm{SE}(\hat{\beta}_j)$ is the standard error of $\hat{\beta}_j$. Under the null hypothesis that $\beta_j = 0$, W^2 has a chi-square distribution with 1 degree of freedom.

A $100(1 - \alpha\%)$ CI for β_j is given by

$$\hat{\beta}_j \pm z_{1-\alpha/2} \times \mathrm{SE}(\hat{\beta}_j), \tag{3.69}$$

where $z_{1-\alpha/2}$ is the $100(1 - \alpha/2)$th quantile of the standard normal distribution and $\mathrm{SE}(\hat{\beta}_j)$ is the estimated standard error for the parameter estimate.

Time-dependent covariates are explanatory variables whose value changes over time. For example, for each week that a patient is on the wait list, the weekly number of direct admissions varies. Also, in studying the effect of surgery on perioperative mortality, it would be necessary to evaluate a time-dependent indicator for surgery. It is relatively easy to incorporate time-dependent covariates into a Cox regression model. First, suppose that there is one time-dependent covariate that is an indicator for some event. Let $\lambda_1(t)$ be the hazard of the outcome event before the time-dependent event occurs, and let $\lambda_2(t)$ be the hazard after the time-dependent event occurs. Incorporating this time-dependent indicator into the model is based on the assumption that the hazard for patients who experienced the outcome after the time-dependent event is proportional to the hazard of patients who did not experience the time-dependent event. The relation between these hazards, given a particular set of covariates, x, is defined as follows:

$$\lambda_2(t|x) = \begin{cases} \lambda_1(t|x), & t < \text{time of intermediate event} \\ \lambda_1(t|x)\text{HR}, & t \geq \text{time of intermediate event}, \end{cases} \tag{3.70}$$

where HR is the hazard ratio associated with the time-dependent event.

An indicator variable, $x_0(t)$, which changes from 0 to 1 at the time of the event, is used to model the time-dependent event. The Cox regression to be estimated is

$$\lambda_0(t)\exp\{\beta_0 x_0(t) + \beta'x\} = \begin{cases} \lambda_0(t)\exp\{\beta'x\}, & t < \text{time of intermediate event} \\ \lambda_0(t)\exp\{\beta_0 + \beta'x\}, & t \geq \text{time of intermediate event}, \end{cases} \tag{3.71}$$

with an unspecified baseline hazard $\lambda_0(t)$ and regression coefficients β_0 corresponding to the time-dependent covariate and β corresponding to the fixed covariates.

In general, suppose there are m time-dependent covariates, which may be binary indicators or continuous variables. Then the Cox regression model in equation 3.66 becomes [3]

$$\lambda_i(t) = \lambda_0(t)\exp\{\beta_1 x_{i1}(t) + \cdots + \beta_m x_{im}(t)\}, \tag{3.72}$$

where $x_{ij}(t)$ is the value of covariate j at time t for patient i. Time-dependent covariates are a convenient way to include information on changes in the patient's and the system's status at any time before and including time t. For example, it may represent the number of direct admissions during week t or it may represent the total number of direct admissions up until week t. Note that models may include both fixed and time-dependent covariates. For fixed covariates, the value of the covariate remains the same across time (that is, $x_{ij}(t) = x_{ij}(0)$ for all t). The regression parameters are estimated via maximum partial likelihood techniques.

Interpretation

The regression coefficients in the Cox model (equation 3.66) quantify the association between the explanatory variables and the hazard of an event. The regression estimates are related to HRs, a familiar measure of comparison described in section 3.3.3. For a binary explanatory variable x_j, for which the reference category is coded as 0, the exponential of the estimate $\hat{\beta}_j$

$$\widehat{\text{HR}} = \exp\{\hat{\beta}_j\}, \tag{3.73}$$

produces the HR that compares the hazard of an event in patients with $x_j = 1$ with the hazard of the event in patients with $x_j = 0$. For example, when the variable x_j represents priority group with a value of 1 for a high-priority patient and a value of 0 for a low-priority patient, the HR greater than 1 indicates higher hazard in higher-priority patients. In general, if HR is 1, there is no difference in the hazard of the event, and if HR is less than 1, the hazard is lower. An approximate $100(1 - \alpha)\%$ CI for this HR is

$$\exp\{\hat{\beta}_j \pm z_{1-\alpha/2} \times \mathrm{SE}(\hat{\beta}_j)\}\,, \tag{3.74}$$

which is not symmetric around the point estimate.

The HR associated with δ-unit increase in continuous variable x_j is estimated by

$$\widehat{\mathrm{HR}} = \exp\{\hat{\beta}_j \times \delta\}\,, \tag{3.75}$$

and its corresponding $100(1 - \alpha)\%$ CI is given

$$\exp\{\hat{\beta}_j \times \delta \pm z_{1-\alpha/2} \times \delta \times \mathrm{SE}(\hat{\beta}_j)\}. \tag{3.76}$$

This HR compares the hazard of the event between groups of patients with values of the continuous variable that differ by δ units. Typically, δ is taken to be 1, such that the change in hazard occurs for every unit increase of the continuous variable. For example, if the variable x_j represents the size of a wait list at registration and $\delta = 1$, then $e^{\hat{\beta}_j}$ represents the factor by which the hazard of the event changes for every additional patient already on the list. The quantity $100 \times |e^{\hat{\beta}_j} - 1|$ estimates the percentage change in hazard for a 1-unit increase in a continuous variable x_j [3]. If x_j is binary, $100 \times |e^{\hat{\beta}_j} - 1|$ estimates the percentage change in hazard in one group relative the reference group. Note that $\log{(\mathrm{HR})} = \log{(e^{\beta})} = \beta$ and $\log(1) = 0$; therefore, testing the hypothesis that HR is different from 1 is equivalent to testing the hypothesis that β is different from 0.

Remarks

The Cox proportional hazards model gets its name from its assumption that hazards are proportional to one another. The proportionality of hazards assumption may be assessed by plotting the logarithm of hazards over time, expecting these curves are parallel. Cox regression is suitable for stratified analysis, in which the baseline hazard is allowed to vary across strata.

In Chapter 9, to measure the treatment-related effect of elective CABG, we used Cox regression with a time-dependent indicator variable (section 3.4.4) that changed from 0 to 1 after surgery [42]. The exponential of the regression coefficient for this variable gave the hazard ratio of death for treated patients relative to those who remained untreated, with a value of less than 1 indicating a reduced hazard resulting from having undergone CABG. We also studied whether survival differed significantly among patients who waited for CABG longer than the target access time (6 weeks for semiurgent procedures and 12 weeks for nonurgent procedure) [70], using a separate model with two time-dependent indicator variables for CABG performed before and after the target time. Point estimates and CIs for HRs were calculated for each urgency group and for the entire cohort. When performing the Cox regression analysis, we stratified on age and sex to avoid the proportionality assumption for these variables.

When more than one event occurs at a certain time, the data are said to be "tied", a situation that is likely to occur with waiting-time data. For example, if time is measured in weeks, multiple patients will experience the event of surgery in the same unit of time (that is, in the same week). In this situation, the methods of analysis should be appropriate to handling ties. Both approximate and exact methods are available for this purpose. When there are more ties than the number of patients still on the wait list, approximate methods give regression estimates that are biased toward 0 [3]. Statistical software can be used to fit Cox regression models, refer to Allison for a practical reference on survival analysis in SAS [3]. This reference includes discussions on using PROC PHREG in SAS to fit Cox regression models. PROC PHREG also allows for time-dependent covariates and tied event times.

If the Cox regression for discrete-time data assumes that the events truly happen at the same time, it is modeling a conditional probability instead of a hazard. Specifically, this approach models the logit of the conditional probability that the patient will experience an event at time t, given that he or she is still on the wait list at that time. It is equivalent to the discrete-time survival regression models discussed in section 3.4.5.

3.4.4 Poisson log-linear regression

In section 3.2.3, we introduced the concept of event rate, and then in section 3.3.3 we defined the rate ratio (RR) as a measure of comparison between groups. In this section, we discuss log-linear regression models that produce RRs to summarize effects, after adjustment for other factors.

Model

The log-linear regression model assumes that the log of the event rate is linearly related to one or more explanatory variables [52]:

$$\log \lambda_i = \alpha + \beta_1 x_{i1} + \cdots + \beta_m x_{im} , \qquad (3.77)$$

where λ_i is the event rate for patient i, and x_{ij} is the value of variable j for patient i. When the number of events is assumed to follow a Poisson distribution and the event rate is constant over the follow-up time, this model is called Poisson regression.

As discussed in section 3.2.3, the event rate is a ratio of the number of events to the total waiting time. Equation 3.77 can also be expressed for the expected number events [52]:

$$\log \mu_i = \alpha + \beta_1 x_{i1} + \cdots + \beta_m x_{im} + \log(t_i) , \qquad (3.78)$$

where μ_i is the expected number of events for patient i, t_i is the waiting time for patient i, and $\log(t_i)$ is referred to as the "offset." Note that the log link restricts the expected number of events to values greater than 0.

The maximum likelihood method is used to estimate the model parameters for a given set of covariates using the Poisson likelihood function as follows [52]

$$L(\alpha, \beta_1, \ldots, \beta_m) = \prod_{i=1}^{n} \frac{\mu_i^{y_i} e^{\mu_i}}{y_i!} , \qquad (3.79)$$

where y_i is a Poisson-distributed random variable for the number of events and μ_i is defined in 3.78. In practice, statistical programs, such as PROC GENMOD in SAS can be used to obtain the parameter estimates.

Interpretation

The regression coefficients in the Poisson model (equation 3.78) quantify association between the event rate and the explanatory variables. The regression estimates are used to obtained RRs; and both crude and adjusted RRs can be estimated with Poisson regression models. For a binary explanatory variable, x_j, for which one category is coded as 1 and the reference category is coded as 0, the exponential of the estimate $\hat{\beta}_j$,

$$\widehat{\mathrm{RR}} = \exp\{\hat{\beta}_j\} \,, \tag{3.80}$$

yields the estimated RR that compares the event rate among patients for whom $x_j = 1$ with the rate of the event among patients for whom $x_j = 0$. For example, when variable x_j represents registration period with a value of 1 for reduced-funding years, the RR less than 1 indicates the lower rate for the reduced-funding years relative to the standard year. If RR is 1, there is no difference in the event rate, and if RR is greater than 1, the event rate is greater. An approximate $100(1-\alpha)\%$ CI for this RR is

$$\exp\{\hat{\beta}_j \pm z_{1-\alpha/2} \times \mathrm{SE}(\hat{\beta}_j)\} \,, \tag{3.81}$$

which is not symmetric around the point estimate.

For a continuous variable, using the maximum likelihood estimate $\hat{\beta}_j$, the effect of increase in value by δ units is estimated by

$$\widehat{\mathrm{RR}} = \exp\{\hat{\beta}_j \times \delta\} \,, \tag{3.82}$$

and by its approximate $100(1-\alpha)\%$ CI

$$\exp\{\hat{\beta}_j \times \delta \pm z_{1-\alpha/2} \times \delta \times \mathrm{SE}(\hat{\beta}_j)\} \,. \tag{3.83}$$

This RR compares the event rate between groups of patients with values of the continuous variable that differ by δ units. If δ is taken to be 1, the change in the event rate is quantified for every unit increase of the variable. For example, if the variable x_j represents the volume of emergency referrals and $\delta = 1$, then $\exp\{\hat{\beta}_j\}$ represents the factor by which the event rate changes for every emergency admission.

The quantity $100 \times |e^{\hat{\beta}_j} - 1|$ estimates the percentage change in rate associated with the 1-unit increase in a continuous variable x_j. If x_j is binary, $100 \times |e^{\hat{\beta}_j} - 1|$ yields the percentage change in rate in one group compared with the reference group.

Remarks

To determine whether the admission rate is constant over the time that patients spend on the wait list, one can test the null hypothesis that the waiting-time distribution is exponential. The rationale is that a constant rate corresponds to an exponential distribution [53].

In Part II, we use Poisson log-linear regression to analyze the relation between the weekly rate of elective vascular surgery and priority group. Using RRs, we compare the rates of surgery between priority groups, finding, for example, that the weekly rate of surgery was 1.7 times higher for priority 2 patients than for priority 3 patients.

Note that $\log(\mathrm{RR}) = \log(e^\beta) = \beta$ and $\log(1) = 0$; therefore, testing the hypothesis that RR is different from 1 is equivalent to testing the hypothesis that β is different from 0.

3.4.5 Discrete-time regression

Discrete-time regression models the relation between time to an event and one or more explanatory variables, when many events could occur at the same time. For example, scheduling patients for surgery provides a weekly opportunity for hospital admission. Measured as the number of service-scheduling cycles, waiting time is therefore inherently discrete and is best measured as the number of new scheduling cycles from registration to admission. Therefore, a key feature of waiting-time data from surgical service is that the scheduling cycle is the unit of analysis. Because scheduling is done weekly, the waiting period is computed as the number of calendar weeks between registration and admission. For those removed from the wait list before admission, waiting time is the number of calendar weeks from registration to removal. In this section, we introduce two regression models that can be used to quantify adjusted effects of study factors when time to event is discrete.

It is common practice in regression analysis of discrete times to perform a pooled analysis of the logistic regression models developed for each time unit of follow-up, treating consecutive periods of observation as ordered strata (see Allison [2]). For each wait-list week t, the regression model is defined by three elements: (1) the indicator variable δ_{it}, which is set to 1 if patient i, who was still on the wait list just before week t, experienced an event of interest and otherwise is set to 0; (2) the probability of the event

$$p_{it} = \Pr(\delta_{it} = 1 \mid x_{i1}, \ldots, x_{im}), \tag{3.84}$$

which is the conditional probability of the event in week t, given that it did not occur in preceding weeks and given the explanatory variables $x_{i1}, \ldots, x_{im}$; and (3) a link function that relates the probability p_{it} to a linear function of the variables $\alpha_t + \beta_1 x_{i1} + \ldots + \beta_m x_{im}$, where α_t characterizes the event rate at week t in the reference group and β_j, $j = 1, \ldots, m$ are regression coefficients.

In the next sections, we consider two common link functions, the logit function and the complementary log-log function, which allow for indicator variables that code the ordered strata to be included in the set of explanatory variables .

Proportional odds model

As its name suggests, the proportional odds model assumes that the odds of an event in one group are proportional to the odds of the event in another group. Let p_{1t} be the conditional probability of the event at time t in group 1, and let p_{0t} be the conditional probability of the event at time t in group 0, the reference group. The proportional odds model then is formulated as follows

$$\frac{p_{1t}}{1 - p_{1t}} = e^\beta \frac{p_{0t}}{1 - p_{0t}}, \tag{3.85}$$

where e^β is the proportionality constant. Applying a log transformation to equation 3.85 gives the basic form of the proportional odds model with one regression coefficient representing group 1:

$$\log\left(\frac{p_{1t}}{1 - p_{1t}}\right) = \alpha_t + \beta, \tag{3.86}$$

the intercept α_t is the log odds of the event at time t in the reference group.

Applying the logit link to relate the conditional probabilities of the event to a linear function of several covariates results in a multivariable proportional odds model:

$$\log\left(\frac{p_{it}}{1 - p_{it}}\right) = \alpha_t + \beta_1 x_{i1} + \cdots + \beta_m x_{im}, \tag{3.87}$$

where β_j is a regression coefficient associated with covariate j. Although it looks similar to the logistic regression model (equation 3.57), this model is fundamentally different because indicator variables that code the consecutive units of follow-up time are included to model the event odds over time.

The parameters of the proportional odds model can be estimated by the maximum likelihood method. The likelihood function for the proportional odds model is

$$L(\alpha_t, \beta_1, \ldots, \beta_m) = \prod_{i=1}^{n} \left(\frac{p_{it_i}}{1 - p_{it_i}} \right)^{\delta_{it}} \prod_{\{j | t_j \le t_i\}} (1 - p_{it_j}), \tag{3.88}$$

where each week of follow-up is assumed to represent an independent period of observation and is included separately for each subject, and $p_{it} = (1 + \exp\{-(\alpha_t + \beta_1 x_{i1} + \cdots + \beta_m x_{im})\})^{-1}$.

Time-dependent covariates can also be incorporated into proportional odds models. With time-dependent covariates, the discrete-time regression model with the logit link function becomes

$$\log \left(\frac{p_{it}}{1 - p_{it}} \right) = \alpha_t + \beta_1 x_{i1}(t) + \cdots + \beta_m x_{im}(t), \tag{3.89}$$

where $x_{ij}(t)$ is the value of covariate j for patient i at time t [2]. Note that the regression coefficients do not change over time.

For analysis of waiting-time data, we consider consecutive weeks on the wait list as independent periods of observation, each included in the data set separately for each patient in a synthetic cohort. The effects of the explanatory variables on the odds of an event of interest are assumed to be constant over consecutive wait-list weeks. Therefore, the regression coefficients in the proportional odds model (equation 3.87) can be interpreted as the log of common ORs. In the same manner as for the logistic regression, the exponential of the estimate $\hat{\beta}_j$ yields the estimated OR of two groups for a binary explanatory variable, and the estimated OR associated with 1-unit increase in a continuous variable; see the Interpretation section for logistic regression coefficients in section 3.4.2.

In a simple case of a constant event rate for all weeks (that is, $\alpha_t = \alpha$) and one indicator variable representing the comparison group, the weekly probability of the event is $(1 + \exp\{-\alpha\})^{-1}$ in the reference group and $(1 + \exp\{-(\alpha + \beta)\})^{-1}$ in the comparison group.

For model 3.89 it is assumed that the effects of time-dependent covariates are constant over time. For example, one direct admission during a patient's 1st week on the wait list is assumed to have the same effect as one direct admission arriving during the patient's 10th week on the list. Therefore, the regression coefficients associated with the time-dependent covariates in model 3.89 can be converted into a similar manner.

In Chapter 6, we use the proportional odds model to evaluate the combined effect of volume of direct admissions on the surgery rate among patients awaiting elective CABG. In multivariable analysis we adjust for age, sex, comorbidity, calendar period of registration, and hospital. For the direct admissions, we interpret the odds ratio as a change in the weekly odds of elective surgery associated with one additional surgery performed immediately after angiography.

Complementary log-log model

The complementary log-log model is the discrete-time version of the proportional hazards model [93, 2]. It is based on the assumption that the conditional probability of no event at time t in one group is the same as the conditional probability of no event at time t in another group to a fixed power. Let p_{1t} and p_{0t} be the conditional probability of an event at time t for group 1 and group 0, respectively. Group 0 is considered the reference group. The complementary log-log model then assumes that for all consecutive times $t = 1, 2, \ldots$ the conditional probabilities of no event in the two groups are related by a fixed power:

$$(1 - p_{1t}) = (1 - p_{0t})^{e^{\beta}} , \qquad (3.90)$$

where e^{β} is some fixed constant. Applying the log-log transformation to equation 3.90 gives the basic form of the complementary log-log model with one explanatory variable for the comparison group:

$$\log(-\log(1 - p_{1t})) = \alpha_t + \beta , \qquad (3.91)$$

where α_t characterizes the hazard of the event at time t in the reference group. Applying the complementary log-log link to relate the conditional probabilities of an event to a linear function of several covariates results in a multivariable regression [93]:

$$\log(-\log(1 - p_{it})) = \alpha_t + \beta_1 x_{i1} + \cdots + \beta_m x_{im} . \qquad (3.92)$$

The parameters of the complementary log-log regression are estimated by the maximum likelihood procedure used for generalized linear models because the time to event has the same likelihood function as a sequence of Bernoulli trials with probability of success p_{it} [2]. The likelihood function for observations consistent with the complementary log-log model is

$$L(\alpha_t, \beta_1, \ldots, \beta_m) = \prod_{i=1}^{n} \left(\frac{p_{it_i}}{1 - p_{it_i}} \right)^{\delta_{it}} \prod_{\{j|t_j \leq t_i\}} (1 - p_{it_j}) , \qquad (3.93)$$

where each week of follow-up is assumed to represent an independent period of observation and is included separately for each subject, and $p_{it} = 1 - \exp\{-\exp\{\alpha_t + \beta_1 x_{i1} + \cdots + \beta_m x_{im}\}\}$. Using the regression estimates, it is possible to derive the HRs to assess the difference among the groups or percentage change associated with an increase in a continuous explanatory variable in the same manner as a for proportional hazards model [3]; see the Interpretation section in 3.4.3.

With time-dependent covariates, the discrete-time regression model with complementary log-log link function in equation 3.92 becomes

$$\log(-\log(1 - p_{it})) = \alpha_t + \beta_1 x_{i1}(t) + \cdots + \beta_m x_{im}(t) , \qquad (3.94)$$

where $x_{ij}(t)$ is the value of covariate j for patient i at time t [93]. It is assumed that the effects of time-dependent covariates do no change over time, so the regression coefficients are constant. Therefore the corresponding regression estimates can be converted into HRs; refer to the Interpretation section in 3.4.3 for further details.

In a simple case of a constant event rate for all weeks (that is, $\alpha_t = \alpha$) and one indicator variable representing the comparison group, the weekly probability of the event is $1 - \exp\{-\exp\{\alpha\}\}$ in the reference group and $1 - \exp\{-\exp\{\alpha + \beta\}\}$ in the comparison group. It is important to note that the model expressed by equation 3.94 is population-based, with the coefficients β representing the average effects of covariates among those at risk. The model is therefore applicable to grouped data.

In Chapter 6, we use a discrete-time regression model with complementary log-log link to express the admission rate for vascular surgery in one wait-list size group relative to that in another group. In a multivariable analysis, the association between the length of wait list at registration and wait to surgery is measured by relative rate of admission adjusted for type of procedure, age, sex, and calendar period of registration.

Remarks

Unlike the proportional odds model, the complementary log-log model assumes that the waiting times are truly continuous, but have been grouped into intervals. Therefore, the regression parameters being estimated with this model have a relative risk interpretation [3].

Both the logit and the complementary log-log link transform probabilities, which range from 0 to 1, to quantities that range from negative infinity to positive infinity. The logit link is symmetric. Therefore, modeling the probability of an event or modeling the probability of no event will simply result in regression coefficients of opposite signs. In contrast, the complementary log-log link is asymmetric. Therefore, modeling the probability of an event and no event will yield regression coefficients of different magnitudes. In contrast to the Cox regression, discrete time regressions also yield estimates of baseline probabilities.

In the analysis of data with time-dependent covariates, patient-level data are converted into patient-time data. In contrast to the patient-level data set, in which each row represents one patient, the patient-time data set consists of one row for each week that the patient spent on the list. A patient who was on the list for 5 weeks would therefore be represented by five rows of data in the patient-time data set. PROC GENMOD in SAS can handle time-dependent covariates for discrete-time regression presented in the patient-time format.

3.4.6 Regression for pseudovalues of cumulative incidence functions

In section 3.2.5, we introduced the cumulative incidence function (CIF) as the time-dependent, marginal probability that an event will occur at or before a certain waiting time in the competing-risks setting. Methods for comparing CIFs between groups were discussed in section 3.3.5. In this section, we describe a regression model for quantifying the adjusted effect of study variables on the CIF. Klein and Andersen [64] proposed an estimation procedure for obtaining the effects of covariates on the CIF for each competing event separately. This approach is based on using regression analysis of pseudovalues for the estimator of the CIF [9].

Model

Because the CIF represents probabilities over time, the proportional odds model is a natural choice for directly relating two CIFs [39]:

$$\frac{F_c(t \mid \text{group 1})}{1 - F_c(t \mid \text{group 1})} = e^{\beta} \frac{F_c(t \mid \text{group 0})}{1 - F_c(t \mid \text{group 0})} \,, \tag{3.95}$$

where $F_c(t \mid \text{group 1})$ and $F_c(t \mid \text{group 0})$ are CIFs of event c for group 1 and group 0, and e^{β} is the proportionality constant. The adjusted effect of a factor on the CIF of the event can be estimated by means of a multivariable logistic regression that models the logit of $F(t \mid \boldsymbol{x}_i)$ as a linear function of covariates $\boldsymbol{x}_i = (x_{i1}, \ldots, x_{ip})'$ for all times $t = 1, \ldots, K$:

$$\log\left(\frac{F(t \mid \boldsymbol{x}_i)}{1 - F(t \mid \boldsymbol{x}_i)}\right) = \alpha_t + \beta' \boldsymbol{x}_i \,, \tag{3.96}$$

where α_t is the logit of the CIF at time t in the reference group; $\beta = (\beta_1, \ldots, \beta_m)'$ is a vector of regression coefficients associated with the covariates; the event-type subscript is suppressed for ease of notation. Note that this model implies that the effects of explanatory variables do not change over time [9, 64].

Klein and Andersen proposed a regression analysis with pseudovalues of the CIF as the outcome. For each subject a series of pseudovalues is estimated. These pseudovalues may be thought of as representing the observed CIF for the subject. Specifically, we let $\hat{F}(t)$ be the estimated CIF based on the observation of n subjects over K time points $t_1, \ldots, t_K$. For subject i, the pseudovalue of the CIF at time t is defined as follows

$$\hat{\theta}_{it} = n\hat{F}(t) - (n-1)\hat{F}^{(i)}(t) , \tag{3.97}$$

where $\hat{F}^{(i)}(t)$ is the estimated CIF modified by removing subject i. In the absence of censoring (that is, all subjects experience one of the competing events during follow-up), the pseudovalues of the CIF have some noteworthy properties. First, for each subject, these pseudovalues correspond to a series of binary variables equal to 0 before and 1 at or after the event of interest (that is, $\hat{\theta}_{it} = 1$, if time to event is greater than or equal to t, 0 otherwise). Second, for a given time, the average of the pseudovalues across subjects corresponds to the value of the CIF at that time, that is,

$$n^{-1} \sum_{i=1}^{n} \hat{\theta}_{it} = \hat{F}(t) . \tag{3.98}$$

Third, when there is no censoring, the pseudovalues are independent; when there is censoring, they are approximately independent [64]. Using the pseudovalues the parameters of the CIF regression model (equation 3.96) are estimated then by generalized estimating equations approach to adjust for subject-level correlation between the pseudovalues [72, 37].

Let $\hat{\theta}_i = (\hat{\theta}_{it})'$ be the estimated vector of pseudovalues across time for subject i and $\mu_i(\gamma) = (\mu(\alpha_t + \beta'x_i))'$ be the $K \times 1$ vector of the corresponding mean function for model 3.96 presented as follows

$$\mu(\alpha_t + \beta'x_i) = (1 + \exp\{-(\alpha_t + \beta'x_i)\})^{-1} . \tag{3.99}$$

The estimating equations take the form

$$\sum_{i=1}^{n} \nabla\mu_i V_i^{-1}(\hat{\theta}_i - \mu_i(\gamma)) = 0 , \tag{3.100}$$

where $\nabla\mu_i$ is the $(K + p) \times K$ matrix of the partial derivatives of μ by γ and V_i is the $K \times K$ working covariance matrix of the pseudovalues for subject i.

The working weight matrix may be fixed and estimated as a product–moment correlation matrix among the pseudovalues of the CIF. Each element of the covariance matrix V_i is given by

$$\hat{v}_{hl} = \frac{1}{n} \sum_{i=1}^{n} (\hat{\theta}_{ih} - \bar{\theta}_h)(\hat{\theta}_{il} - \bar{\theta}_l) , \tag{3.101}$$

where $\bar{\theta}_h = \frac{1}{n}\sum_{i=1}^{n} \hat{\theta}_{ih}$. The independence of the pseudovalues across subjects is addressed by Andersen et al [9], and the independence of the pseudovalues within subjects is addressed by Klein et al [64].

Interpretation

The regression coefficients in the CIF pseudovalue model (equation 3.96) quantify the effect of explanatory variables on the CIF. In this model the effects of the explanatory variables on the logit-transformed CIF are assumed to be constant over time. Since the CIF represents a series of probabilities, we can interpret the exponential of the regression coefficients as the OR of two groups for a binary explanatory variable, and the OR associated with a 1-unit increase in a continuous variable; see the Interpretation section for logistic regression coefficients in section 3.4.2. Klein argued that when studying events in a competing-risks setting, the results for all risks should be reported [64].

Remarks

The logit function is one possible link function for relating the pseudovalues of the CIF to the explanatory variables. Another possible link function is complementary log-log [64]. When using a logit or complementary log-log link, the estimated regression coefficients are approximately unbiased, with as few as five time points. Klein recommended using pseudovalues at 10 or more time points for good estimates [64]. In practice, statistical programs, like PROC GENMOD in SAS, can be used to obtain parameter estimates.

In addition to Klein and Andersen, others have proposed regression models related to the CIF [64]. Fine and Gray proposed a method for modeling the subhazard [40, 91]. Bryant and Dignam discussed semiparametric models for the CIF [21].

Waiting-time Studies

Overview of waiting times and other variables

4.1 Introduction

In Part II of this book, we present various analyses of waiting-time data for elective vascular surgery, chole-cystectomy, and coronary artery bypass grafting, all based on the data sets described in Chapter 2. In the current chapter, we define and categorize the outcomes, study variables, and confounders for each of the three data sets used in the subsequent analyses. Then, in Chapters 5 through 10, we address the questions on access to elective care posed in Chapter 1, using the statistical methods presented in Chapter 3.

4.2 Elective vascular surgery

4.2.1 Waiting times

We studied prospectively the waiting times experienced by a cohort of patients registered on wait lists for elective vascular surgery to be provided by a single team of specialists at an acute care hospital in Ontario. A detailed description of the elective vascular surgery data is given in Chapter 2. SAS Code B.1 and B.2 (see Appendix) shows how we used a DATA step to prepare the analytical data set. This data set is used in the analyses and SAS examples presented throughout the remainder of this book. The following procedures were considered: repair of abdominal aortic aneurysm, carotid endarterectomy, peripheral vascular bypass surgery and other procedures for peripheral vascular disease involving blood supply to the legs, or vascular access for dialysis. For each patient, waiting time was calculated in calendar weeks from registration to surgery or to removal from the list without surgery. The date of the surgeon's letter to the referring primary care physician regarding acceptance for surgery served as the date of registration on the list.

In the majority of our analyses, we used discrete-time survival analysis because waiting time is inherently discrete and is best measured by the number of weekly operating room schedules [107].

4.2.2 Confounders

Multivariable models were used to control for differences in patient characteristics and important confounders (summarized in Table 2.5). In one analysis, we studied two calendar periods in which patients were accepted for surgery: period 1 covered the time before March 31, 1997, and period 2, the time from that date forward. A decrease in operating time from 3.0 in period 1 to 2.6 days per week in period 2, because of a decrease in the number of anesthetists, raised concerns about differences in access to elective surgery between the periods.

4.2.3 Wait-list size

For each calendar week during the study, the demand for surgery was characterized according to the queue length and the batch size of arrivals. For each patient, list size was calculated by a simple census of patients with higher or equal queuing priority already on the list at the time of registration. Patients contributed one count to the wait-list size for each week on the list, except the week of arrival. As operations are routinely scheduled 1 week in advance, patients who underwent surgery were considered to have been removed from the wait list in the calendar week preceding their admission dates. Patients whose operations were deferred indefinitely contributed to the queue length for 52 weeks after their registration. For each patient, the batch size of arrivals was the count of patients with higher or equal queuing priority registered on the list in the same week.

List size at registration was categorized by clearance time, that is, a hypothetical time within which the list could be cleared at a maximum weekly service capacity if there were no new arrivals. This time was calculated as the number of patients on the list divided by the average weekly number of removals from the list. Given the capacity level of 5 operations a week in this service, 0–4 patients on the list corresponded to a clearance time of 1 week; 5–20, to 1 month; and 21 or more, to more than 1 month. Similarly, batch sizes of arrivals were divided into categories of 1–4 and 5 or more.

To investigate the effect of total demand during a certain week, we divided patients into six strata according to a combination of list-size and batch-size categories: list < 5 and batch < 5, list < 5 and batch $\geq$5, list 5–20 and batch < 5, list 5–20 and batch $\geq$5, list $\geq$21 and batch < 5, and list $\geq$21 and batch $\geq$5.

4.3 Elective cholecystectomy

4.3.1 Waiting times

A detailed description of the elective cholecystectomy data is given in Chapter 2. SAS Code B.5 (see Appendix) shows how we used a DATA step to prepare the analytical data set. This data set is used in the analyses and SAS examples presented throughout the remainder of this book. A waiting time based on the number of weeks from the last consultation visit to elective or emergency surgery was calculated for each patient. This approach assumes that the last visit before surgery is the date of the decision to operate [35].

4.3.2 Confounders

Age decade, sex, registration period and the surgeon's annual volume of cholecystectomies were considered potential confounding variables.

4.4 Elective coronary artery bypass surgery

4.4.1 Waiting times

A detailed description of the elective coronary artery bypass grafting data is given in Chapter 2. SAS Code B.3 and B.4 in the Appendix shows how we used a DATA step to prepare the analytical data set. This data set is used in the analyses and SAS examples presented throughout the remainder of this book. The time on the wait list was computed as the number of calendar weeks from registration to surgery, death or removal from the wait list. The date of the surgeon's request to book the operating room served as the date of registration on the wait list. Waiting times were treated as prospective observations that were monitored from registration to the patient's last week on the list.

In the majority of our analyses, we used discrete-time survival analysis because waiting time is inherently discrete and is best measured by the number of weekly operating room schedules [107]. We represented time to event by a sequence of binary variables indicating if the patient experienced the event during a certain wait-list week. The likelihood function of such indicators is defined by conditional probabilities of an event in a certain week among those remaining on the list [2]. To fit a pool of logistic regression models (equation 3.87), it was assumed that binary indicators were independent across patients, as described in Chapter 3.

4.4.2 Waiting outcomes

To identify type of admission for surgery (elective or unplanned emergency), hospital admission and discharge dates, coexisting conditions, and in-hospital deaths, we used a patient's Provincial Health Number to deterministically link the British Columbia Cardiac Registry (BCCR) records to the British Columbia Linked Health Database Hospital Separations File [25]. Unplanned emergency surgeries were identified by the emergency or urgent code for admission from the emergency department or the emergency code for admission from the admitting department after the patient was registered on a surgical wait list. Data on coexisting conditions were retrieved in the form of diagnoses reported in discharge abstracts created during the calendar year before the treatment decision [56]. To identify deaths that did not occur in a hospital, we linked the BCCR records to the British Columbia Linked Health Database Deaths File [117].

4.4.3 Confounders

The existing literature suggests that elderly patients are more likely to undergo revascularization as an urgent procedure [26], that a smaller coronary vessel diameter may account for the higher risk of adverse cardiovascular events in women [87], that coexisting medical conditions may delay open heart surgery [82], that postoperative survival depends on institutional constraints and individual care providers [36], and that changes in practice or supplementary funds may reduce time until surgery [70]. All of these factors were entered into multivariable regressions in our study.

We used multivariable models to control for differences in patient characteristics and significant confounders (summarized in Table 2.3). In particular, we entered two indicator variables, one for any of a specified group of coexisting medical conditions (congestive heart failure, diabetes mellitus, chronic obstructive pulmonary disease, cancer or rheumatoid arthritis [83]) and the other for other coexisting chronic conditions as defined by Romano et al [97]. Presentation without coexisting conditions was the reference category. We also entered an indicator variable for each hospital in the models to obtain regression estimates for the study variables adjusted for possible variations in access management. Hospital 1 was coded as the referent. To assess whether the estimated models were consistent with our data we used the likelihood ratio test.

4.4.4 Wait-list size

For each patient, list size was calculated by a simple census of patients, in the same hospital, with higher or equal queuing priority already on the list at the time of registration. Patients contributed one count to the wait-list size for each week they stayed on the list, except for the week of arrival. As operations are routinely scheduled 1 week in advance, patients who underwent surgery were considered to have been removed from the wait list in the calendar week preceding their admission dates. Patients whose operations were deferred indefinitely contributed to the queue length for 52 weeks after their registration. For each patient, the batch size of arrivals was the count of patients with higher or equal queuing priority registered on the list in the same week.

The wait-list size was categorized by clearance time, that is, a hypothetical time within which the list could be cleared at a maximum weekly service capacity if there were no new arrivals. We categorized wait-list size as less than a week, half a month, a month, or more than one month of clearance time. In three of the four participating hospitals that had a service capacity of 15 operations per week, wait lists of up to 14, 15 to 29, 30 to 59 and more than 60 patients corresponded to clearance time of a week, half a month, a month, and more than one month. In the fourth hospital, which had a service capacity of 25 operations per week, the same clearance times corresponded to up to 24, 25 to 49, 50 to 99 and more than 100 patients on the list. SAS Code B.8 and in the Appendix shows how we used DATA steps to compute list size.

Batch size (the number of new registrations) was categorized as to whether or not it exceeded the weekly number of operating room slots allocated exclusively to patients on the wait lists. We divided batch size values into two categories: (1) 1 to 6 patients at the three hospitals with a service capacity of 15 operations per week and 1 to 12 patients at the fourth hospital; and (2) 7 or more patients at the three hospitals with a service capacity of 15 operations per week and 13 or more patients at the fourth hospital. Similar SAS code for computing list size was used to compute batch size.

The weekly number of direct admissions was treated as a continuous variable.

5

Variation and access probabilities

5.1 Introduction

Whether waiting times vary by chance alone after adjustment for clinical factors, variation in demand, and patient and hospital characteristics remains an important question in health services research on access to surgery. Surprisingly, little attention has been given to the variation in times spent in a single queue. As described in Chapter 1, it is useful to estimate the proportion of patients who are admitted from a wait list within certain time frames after registration. In this chapter, we present results for admission rate and access probabilities according to length of stay on the list.

5.2 What is the variation in time spent waiting for elective surgery?

The objective of this study was to evaluate the variation in time spent on the wait list for elective vascular surgery provided by the same team of specialists, where queuing procedures were uniform (Chapter 2). Compared to our previous analysis in [103], we added patients who were registered on the wait list after 1998.

The study was primarily concerned with the statistical variation in duration of waiting in a queue of patients with equal surgical needs and urgency. We compared the number of weeks required for specified proportions of patients to undergo the operation by sex and age groups. The cumulative probabilities of undergoing surgery within a certain time were estimated using the product-limit method [17], as described in Chapter 3; waiting times were treated as prospective observations that were monitored from registration until the patient's last week on the list. The log-rank test, described in Chapter 3, was used to compare waiting times across groups [18]. SAS Code B.6 (see Appendix) shows a macro we used to estimate event proportions by group.

The average weekly rate of surgery, that is the total number of admissions divided by the total number of patient-weeks of follow-up, was calculated as a measure of the rate of admission within each priority group; see Chapter 3. SAS Code B.7 (see Appendix) shows a macro we used to estimate event rates by group.

Then, the effect size of priority group on the weekly rate of surgery was estimated by means of the Poisson log-linear model (3.78), which yielded the rate ratio (RR) [52], as discussed in Chapter 3. We determined whether the admission rate was constant over the time patients spent on the wait list by testing the null hypothesis that the waiting-time distribution is exponential. The rationale is that a constant rate

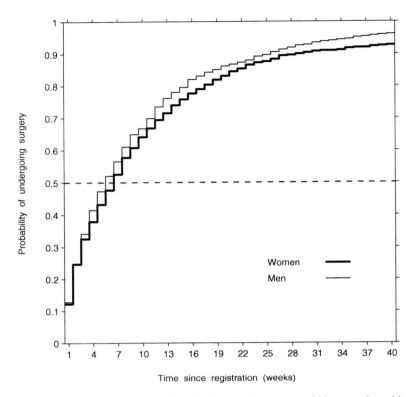

Fig. 5.1. Estimated probability of undergoing elective vascular surgery within a certain waiting time, by sex

corresponds to exponential distribution of waiting times [54]. We used multivariable models to control for differences in age, sex, and registration period.

Among 1916 patients waiting for elective vascular surgery, 1743 (91.0%) received access to surgery. The median waiting time from registration to surgery was 6 weeks (95% CI 6–7). Waiting times were such that 10%, 25%, 75%, and 90% of patients underwent surgery within 1, 3, 14, and 27 weeks from registration. The last 10% of patients waited 5 to 16 weeks, 12 to 25 weeks, 19 to 41 weeks, and 24 to 41 weeks in priority groups 1, 2, 3, and 4, respectively (Table 5.1). The overall average weekly admission rate was 9.7 per 100 patient-weeks (95% CI 9.2–10.1).

There was a difference in access to surgery between men and women, as measured by the log-rank test (test statistic = 5.5, df = 1, $p = 0.02$), with men having a greater chance of surgery within a certain time (Figure 5.1). There was also a difference in access to surgery between age groups, as measured by the log-rank test (test statistic = 37.9, df = 3, $p < 0.0001$), with shorter waiting times for older patients (Figure 5.2).

We estimated the effect of priority group on weekly admission rates using a Poisson log-linear regression model (equation 3.77). The expected number of events, μ, was modeled as a log-linear function of priority group as defined in SAS Code B.1 (see Appendix):

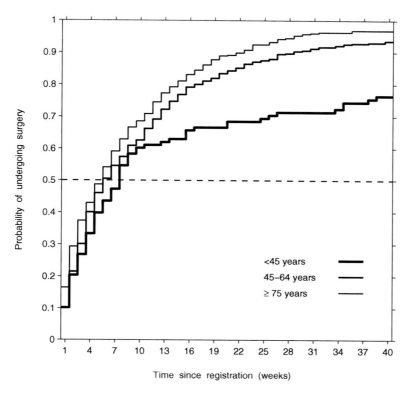

Fig. 5.2. Estimated probability of undergoing elective vascular surgery within a certain waiting time, by age

$$\log \mu = \alpha + \beta_1 \texttt{pr1} + \beta_2 \texttt{pr2} + \beta_3 \texttt{pr3} + \beta_4 \texttt{pr4} + \log(\texttt{wait})$$

where `pr1` is 1 for priority 1 and 0 otherwise, `pr2` is 1 for priority 2 and 0 otherwise, `pr3` is 1 for priority 3 and 0 otherwise, `pr4` is 1 for priority 4 and 0 otherwise, and `wait` is the waiting time in weeks.

SAS Code 5.1 shows how we used PROC GENMOD to estimate the parameters of this model. The GENMOD procedure fits generalized linear models, which are an extension of traditional linear models that allows the population mean to depend on a linear predictor through a nonlinear link function [85]. First, we used a DATA step to create an offset variable. Then we used PROC GENMOD to fit a Poisson regression model (SAS Output 5.1). Relative to priority 5, the parameter estimates decreased with lower urgency: 1.74 (SE = 0.07) for priority 1, 1.02 (SE = 0.09) for priority 2, 0.45 (SE = 0.08) for priority 3, and 0.16 (SE = 0.07) for priority 4. The rate ratios corresponding to SAS Output 5.1 are shown in Table 5.2.

Using a chi-square test, we tested the null hypothesis that weekly probabilities of admission are constant over time spent on wait lists and found that these probabilities were not constant over time (Table 5.2, Figure 5.3). We concluded that when queuing procedures are uniform, the waiting times for access to elective vascular surgery provided by the same team of specialists differ considerably for patients with equal surgical needs and urgency.

SAS Code 5.1: Poisson log-linear regression of weekly admission rates on priority group

```
* create offset variable *;
data admisdat;
  set vasc;
    where wait>0;
    ltime=log(wait);
    admis=0; if status=0 then admis=1;
run;

* Poisson regression *;
proc genmod data=admisdat;
  model admis=pr1 pr2 pr3 pr4 /d=poisson link=log offset=ltime waldci;
run;
```

SAS Output 5.1: Results from Poisson log-linear regression of weekly admission rates on priority group

```
              Analysis Of Parameter Estimates

                          Standard      Wald 95%         Chi-
Parameter   DF  Estimate    Error   Confidence Limits   Square   Pr > ChiSq

Intercept    1   -2.6864   0.0370   -2.7589   -2.6140   5282.72     <.0001
pr1          1    1.7406   0.0690    1.6053    1.8760    635.51     <.0001
pr2          1    1.0194   0.0937    0.8358    1.2030    118.45     <.0001
pr3          1    0.4474   0.0757    0.2990    0.5958     34.91     <.0001
pr4          1    0.1644   0.0691    0.0289    0.2999      5.65      0.0174
Scale        0    1.0000   0.0000    1.0000    1.0000
```

Table 5.1. Characteristics of waiting-time distributions for elective vascular surgery, by sex, age, surgical procedure, and priority group

Factor	No. of patients	Procedures performed, %	Median (95% CI)	10th	25th	75th	90th	Maximum time
Sex								
Women	677	88.8	7 (6–8)	1	3	15	29	41
Men	1239	92.2	6 (5–7)	1	3	13	26	41
Age (years)								
< 45	110	76.4	8 (6–10)	1	3	37	41	41
45–64	518	90.9	6 (5–7)	1	3	15	29	41
65–74	757	92.9	7 (6–7)	1	3	13	24	41
≥ 75	531	91.3	6 (5–7)	1	2	13	23	41
Registration period								
1994–1996	610	90.7	6 (5–6)	1	2	14	27	41
1997–2002	1306	91.1	7 (6–7)	2	3	14	27	41
Procedure								
AAA repair	485	94.6	8 (7–9)	1	3	13	20	41
CEA	411	90.8	10 (8–12)	2	5	19	30	41
PVD surgery	652	87.3	4 (3–4)	1	2	12	37	41
AVF for hemodialysis	368	92.9	5 (5–6)	2	3	10	21	41
Priority								
1 (most urgent)	344	95.6	2	1	1	3	5	16
2	149	95.3	4 (3–5)	1	2	7	12	25
3	247	93.9	7 (6–8)	2	3	12	19	41
4	313	93.9	11 (9–12)	3	6	16	24	41
5 (least urgent)	863	86.4	8 (7–9)	2	4	20	39	41

Abbreviations: CI = confidence interval, AAA = abdominal aortic aneurysm, CEA = carotid endarterectomy,

PVD = peripheral vascular disease, AVF = arteriovenous fistula

Table 5.2. Weekly admission rates for elective vascular surgery, by priority group

Priority	Weekly admission rate*				Crude RR (95% CI)	Test statistic[†]	p value
	Average	(SE)	Minimum	Maximum			
1 (most urgent)	43.5	(2.4)	20.0	45.7	5.7 (5.0–6.5)	82.0	< 0.0001
2	19.9	(1.7)	9.8	30.0	2.8 (2.3–3.3)	8.4	< 0.01
3	10.8	(0.7)	5.9	23.1	1.6 (1.3–1.8)	18.8	< 0.0001
4	8.1	(0.5)	2.6	23.5	1.2 (1.0–1.3)	192.2	< 0.0001
5 (least urgent)	6.9	(0.3)	1.4	10.0	1.0	2.2	0.14

Abbreviations: SE = standard error, RR = rate ratio, CI = confidence interval

*Weekly admission rate was calculated as the number of elective procedures divided by the sum of waiting times (per 100 patient-weeks)

[†] For testing the hypothesis that the waiting time distribution is exponential

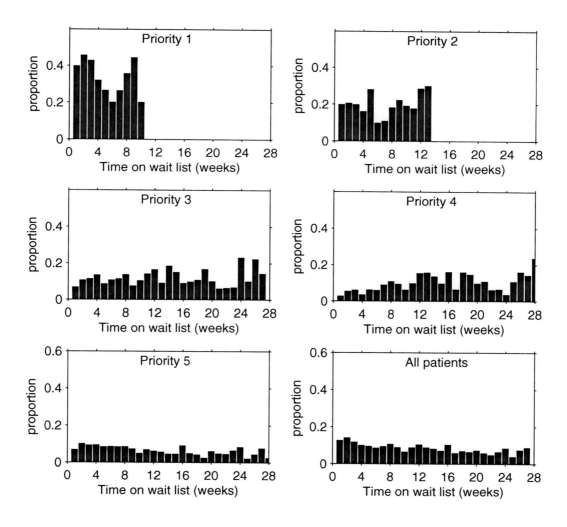

Fig. 5.3. Weekly proportion of elective admissions (that is, conditional probability of admission), by waiting time and priority group

5.3 What is the probability of undergoing surgery within a certain time?

5.3.1 Elective vascular surgery

Previously, we performed a study to evaluate the probability of undergoing elective vascular surgery within a certain time among patients on wait lists, as described in [103]. Here, we updated our analysis by including patients who were registered on the wait list after 1998.

The cumulative probabilities of undergoing surgery within a certain time were estimated using the product-limit method [17], as described in Chapter 3; waiting times were treated as prospective observations that were monitored from registration until the patient's last week on the list.

Of the 1916 cases, 1743 (91.0%) underwent surgery, 71 (3.7%) were still waiting at the end of the follow-up period, and 102 (5.3%) were removed from the list without surgery for a variety of reasons (Table 5.3). Among those who received surgery, the proportions within and beyond recommended times were almost equal (50.9% and 49.1%, respectively). Among those who were removed from the list without having surgery, 31.4% were removed before recommended times expired. The main reason patients waited longer than the recommended times was the length of the wait list (997/1916 or 52.0%).

Table 5.3. Waiting outcomes and scheduling delays for patients registered for elective vascular surgery

Waiting outcomes	n	(%)
Surgery received		
Immediate access	60	(3.1)
Access within recommended times	827	(43.2)
Access beyond recommended times		
Because of the length of the wait list	586	(30.6)
Because of delay in scheduling surgery	270	(14.1)
Surgery not received		
Removed from list before recommended times expired	32	(1.7)
Removed from list after recommended times expired		
Waited because of the length of the wait list	39	(2.0)
Waited because of delay in scheduling surgery	31	(1.6)
Still on the list beyond recommended times		
Because of the length of the wait list	20	(1.0)
Because of delay in scheduling surgery	51	(2.7)

Among patients waiting for elective vascular surgery, there were 1743 procedures over 18 015 patient-weeks. The overall average weekly surgery rate was 9.7 per 100 patient-weeks (95% CI 9.2–10.1).

SAS Code 5.2 shows how we used PROC LIFETEST to estimate the percentiles of waiting time to surgery and the probabilities of surgery within certain times. The LIFETEST procedure computes these estimates by the non-parametric product-limit method. Waiting times were such that 25%, 50%, 75%, and 90% of patients underwent surgery in 3, 6, 14, and 27 weeks, respectively (SAS Output 5.2). The chances of undergoing surgery by 1, 2, 3, 4 and 13 weeks on the list, the target access times, were 0.13, 0.25, 0.34,

0.40, and 0.75, respectively (SAS Output 5.2). The median time to surgery was 6 weeks and the cumulative probability of surgery by 13 weeks from registration was 75% (see Figure 3.1). Therefore, we concluded that patients wait considerably different times for access to elective surgery provided by the same team of specialists.

SAS Code 5.2: Product-limit estimates of waiting time percentiles and cumulative probabilities of admission

```
proc lifetest data=vasc method=km intervals = (1 to 40 by 1);
  where wait>0;
  time wait*status(1 2 3 4 5 6 7 8);
run;
```

SAS Output 5.2: Results from product-limit estimates of cumulative probabilities of admission

The LIFETEST Procedure

Product-Limit Survival Estimates

wait	Survival	Failure	Survival Standard Error	Number Failed	Number Left
0.0000	1.0000	0	0	0	1856
1.0000	0.8745	0.1255	0.00769	233	1623
2.0000	0.7521	0.2479	0.0100	459	1389
3.0000	0.6638	0.3362	0.0110	620	1211
4.0000	0.5978	0.4022	0.0114	740	1086
5.0000	0.5414	0.4586	0.0116	842	979
6.0000	0.4952	0.5048	0.0117	925	891
7.0000	0.4488	0.5512	0.0117	1008	803
8.0000	0.4012	0.5988	0.0115	1093	715
9.0000	0.3657	0.6343	0.0113	1156	650
10.0000	0.3420	0.6580	0.0112	1198	605
11.0000	0.3119	0.6881	0.0109	1251	549
12.0000	0.2794	0.7206	0.0106	1308	490
13.0000	0.2548	0.7452	0.0103	1351	446
14.0000	0.2340	0.7660	0.0100	1387	406
15.0000	0.2175	0.7825	0.00980	1415	369
16.0000	0.1951	0.8049	0.00944	1453	331
17.0000	0.1839	0.8161	0.00924	1472	310
18.0000	0.1713	0.8287	0.00901	1493	285
19.0000	0.1604	0.8396	0.00879	1511	265
20.0000	0.1488	0.8512	0.00855	1530	245
21.0000	0.1403	0.8597	0.00836	1544	230
22.0000	0.1336	0.8664	0.00820	1555	219
23.0000	0.1250	0.8750	0.00799	1569	205
24.0000	0.1145	0.8855	0.00771	1586	184

25.0000	0.1101	0.8899	0.00759	1593	175
26.0000	0.1018	0.8982	0.00736	1606	161
27.0000	0.0929	0.9071	0.00709	1620	145
28.0000	0.0884	0.9116	0.00695	1627	137
29.0000	0.0825	0.9175	0.00676	1636	128
30.0000	0.0799	0.9201	0.00667	1640	122
31.0000	0.0746	0.9254	0.00648	1648	112
32.0000	0.0712	0.9288	0.00636	1653	105
33.0000	0.0699	0.9301	0.00631	1655	103
34.0000	0.0671	0.9329	0.00621	1659	99
35.0000	0.0637	0.9363	0.00608	1664	93
36.0000	0.0596	0.9404	0.00592	1670	87
37.0000	0.0582	0.9418	0.00586	1672	84
38.0000	0.0548	0.9452	0.00571	1677	79
39.0000	0.0526	0.9474	0.00562	1680	74
40.0000	0.0505	0.9495	0.00553	1683	71
41.0000*	.	.	.	1683	0

NOTE: The marked survival times are censored observations.

Summary Statistics for Time Variable wait

Quartile Estimates

| | Point | 95% Confidence Interval | |
Percent	Estimate	[Lower	Upper)
75	14.0000	13.0000	15.0000
50	6.0000	6.0000	7.0000
25	3.0000	2.0000	3.0000

Mean	Standard Error
10.2801	0.2520

NOTE: The mean survival time and its standard error were
underestimated because the largest observation was censored and
the estimation was restricted to the largest event time.

Summary of the Number of Censored and Uncensored Values

| | | | Percent |
Total	Failed	Censored	Censored
1856	1683	173	9.32

5.3.2 Elective coronary artery bypass grafting

We performed a study to evaluate the variation in time spent on the wait lists for coronary artery bypass grafting (CABG) among patients awaiting elective surgery, as described in [70] (Chapter 2). Here, we limited the analysis to patients who were registered for first-time isolated CABG. The cumulative probabilities of undergoing surgery within a certain time were estimated using the product-limit method [17]; waiting times were treated as prospective observations that were monitored from registration until the patient's last week on the list, as described in Chapter 3.

Among patients awaiting elective CABG, there were 7654 procedures over 136 746 patient-weeks. Among the 8728 patients (94.9%) who were removed from the list by 52 weeks, 7654 received planned surgery, 314 underwent unplanned emergency surgery, 91 died, 173 became unfit for surgery, 104 declined surgery, 98 were transferred to another surgeon or hospital, 23 received other surgery, and 188 were removed for other reasons (Table 5.4). The overall average weekly surgery rate was 5.6 per 100 patient-weeks (95% CI 5.5–5.7). The waiting times were such that 25%, 50%, 75%, and 90% of patients underwent surgery in 5, 12, 23, and 46 weeks, respectively. The chances of undergoing surgery by 3, 6, 12, 25, and 52 weeks on the list were 0.18, 0.31, 0.53, 0.79, and 0.91, respectively (Figure 5.4).

Again, we conclude that there was a considerable variation in delays for surgical revascularization in a regional healthcare system. It remains to be examined whether events related to the wait-list management, for example, delays in scheduling operations and surgery cancellations, affect the waiting time after adjustment for urgency and comorbidity status.

Table 5.4. Waiting outcomes at 52 weeks since registration for elective coronary artery bypass grafting, by priority group

Waiting outcomes	All patients n (%)	Urgent n (%)	Semiurgent n (%)	Nonurgent n (%)
Surgery at planned date*				
Immediate access	253 (2.8)	137 (21.2)	108 (1.7)	7 (0.4)
Within recommended time	2528 (27.5)	0 (0.0)	1981 (30.6)	547 (27.9)
Beyond recommended time	4833 (52.5)	433 (67.0)	3513 (54.2)	852 (43.5)
Removal from wait list				
Unplanned emergency surgery	314 (3.4)	50 (7.7)	205 (3.2)	57 (2.9)
Died while waiting	91 (0.1)	4 (0.6)	54 (0.8)	26 (1.3)
Became unfit for surgery	173 (1.9)	3 (0.5)	88 (1.4)	78 (4.0)
Patient request	187 (2.0)	2 (0.3)	130 (2.0)	51 (2.6)
Transferred or moved	98 (1.1)	2 (0.3)	62 (0.1)	31 (1.6)
Other surgery	23 (0.3)	1 (0.2)	13 (0.2)	8 (0.4)
Other reason	188 (2.0)	9 (1.4)	117 (1.8)	57 (2.9)
Still on wait list	471 (5.1)	5 (0.8)	210 (3.2)	245 (12.5)

* Additional 40 (0.4%) with unknown priority underwent surgery between 1 and 12 weeks

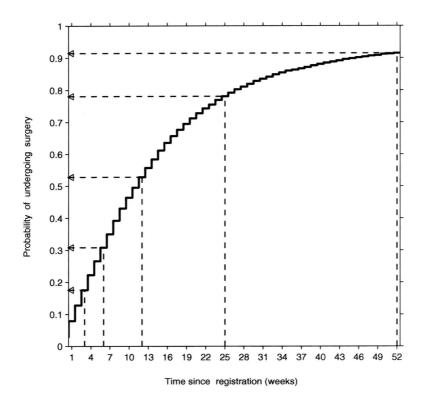

Fig. 5.4. Probability of undergoing elective coronary artery bypass grafting within a certain waiting time, as estimated by the product-limit method. Arrows show probability of undergoing surgery by 3, 6, 12, 25, and 52 weeks.

6

Factors influencing waiting times

6.1 Introduction

In Chapter 1, we described the following factors that affect time to surgery: level of demand, hospital resources, wait-list management, and patient characteristics. In this chapter, we present the results of several studies investigating the relations between factors within and outside surgical care and waiting times for surgery. We show that measuring the proportion of wait-listed patients undergoing treatment within a certain period can clarify the role of these factors in accessing surgical services.

6.2 Does priority affect chances of admission for surgery?

6.2.1 Elective vascular surgery

The objective of this study was to compare the time spent on the wait list for elective vascular surgery by priority group (Chapter 2). Compared to our previous analysis in [103], we added patients who were registered on the wait list after 1998. We compared the number of weeks required for specified proportions of patients to undergo the operation by priority group. The cumulative probabilities of undergoing surgery within a certain time were estimated using the product-limit method [17], as described in Chapter 3; waiting times were treated as prospective observations that were monitored from registration until the patient's last week on the list. The log-rank test, described in Chapter 3, was used to compare waiting times across priority groups [18].

The average weekly rate of surgery, that is, the total number of admissions divided by the total number of patient-weeks of follow-up, was calculated as a measure of the rate of admission within each priority group; see Chapter 3. Then, the effect size of priority group on the weekly rate of surgery was estimated by means of Poisson regression (3.78), which yielded the rate ratio (RR) [52], as discussed in Chapter 3. For this model, in addition to variables coding priority group as in section 5.2, we entered age, sex, and registration period to obtain adjusted rate ratios.

Waiting times varied across priority groups. SAS Code 6.1 shows how we used PROC LIFETEST to evaluate the association between waiting times and priority group. SAS Output 6.1 shows that priority had a major influence on waiting times, with shorter times for higher-priority groups, as measured by the log-rank test and Wilcoxon test. In priority group 5, waiting times were such that 10%, 25%, 50%, 75%, and 90% of the patients underwent surgery in 2, 3, 8, 20, and 39 weeks, respectively. In contrast, half of the patients in priority groups 1, 2, 3, and 4 underwent surgery in 2, 3, 7, and 11 weeks, respectively (Figure 6.1). Patients in higher-priority groups had less than a 30% chance of undergoing surgery within the target access times: 8% of those with priority 1 underwent surgery within 1 week, 17% of those with priority 2 within 2 weeks, 27% of those with priority 3 within 3 weeks, and 16% of those with priority 4 within 4 weeks. Priority 5 patients had a 65% chance of undergoing surgery within 13 weeks, the target access time.

SAS Code 6.1: Comparison of access curves across priority groups

```
proc lifetest data=vasc method=km intervals = (1 to 40 by 1);
  time wait*status(1 2 3 4 5 6 7 8);
  strata urgstat;
run;
```

SAS Output 6.1: Results from comparison of access curves across priority groups

```
              Test  of  Equality  over  Strata

                                       Pr >
    Test        Chi-Square     DF    Chi-Square

    Log-Rank     756.9964       4      <.0001
    Wilcoxon     732.8910       4      <.0001
    -2Log(LR)    640.8100       4      <.0001
```

The surgery rates were greater among higher-priority patients, ranging from 43.5 per 100 patient-weeks for patients with priority 1 to 6.9 per 100 patient-weeks for patients with priority 5 (Table 6.1). Among those who underwent surgery, 48.0% of priority 1 patients did so within target times, whereas only 17.3% of priority 4 patients received timely access (Table 6.2). The odds of surgery within target times were about 5, 3, 2, and 14 times greater for patients with priority 1, 2, 3, and 5, respectively, than for patients with priority 4. The median residual waiting times were longer for lower-priority groups and tended to fluctuate over time (Figure 6.2).

Patients with equal surgical needs spend considerably different times on a wait list to elective surgery provided by the same team of specialists, where queuing procedures are uniform. These variations in waiting times within priority groups suggest that urgency of intervention is not the only factor influencing time spent in a queue for elective surgery.

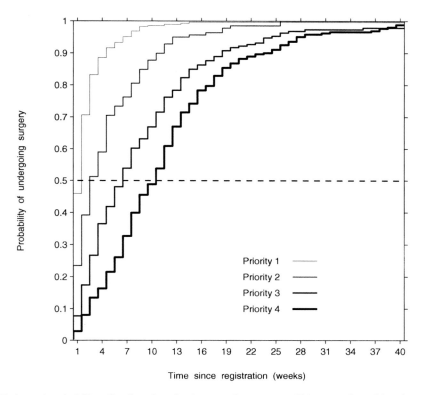

Fig. 6.1. Estimated probability of undergoing elective vascular surgery within a certain waiting time, by priority group

Table 6.1. Relation between priority group and weekly rate of elective vascular surgery, as measured by rate ratios derived from Poisson log-linear regression models

Priority	No. of procedures	Total wait (patient-weeks)	Surgery rate*	(95% CI)	Adjusted RR	(95% CI)
1 (most urgent)	329	757	43.5	(38.8–48.2)	3.62	(3.04–4.30)
2	142	715	19.9	(16.6–23.1)	1.73	(1.40–2.15)
3	232	2149	10.8	(9.4–12.2)	1.00	
4	294	3649	8.1	(7.1–9.0)	0.72	(0.61–0.86)
5 (least urgent)	746	10745	6.9	(6.4–7.4)	0.67	(0.58–0.78)

Abbreviations: CI = confidence interval, RR = rate ratio, adjusted for age, sex, and registration period

* Surgery rate was calculated as the number of elective procedures divided by the sum of waiting times
(per 100 patient-weeks)

Table 6.2. Relation between priority group and probability of undergoing elective vascular surgery within target access time for those who underwent such surgery, as measured by odds ratios derived from logistic regression models

Priority	No. of procedures performed	No. of procedures within TAT	Procedures within TAT, %	90th–100th percentiles (weeks)	OR* (95% CI)
1 (most urgent)	329	158	48.0	5–16	4.5 (3.1–6.6)
2	142	58	40.8	12–26	3.3 (2.1–5.1)
3	232	66	28.4	19–41	1.5 (1.3–2.9)
4	294	51	17.3	24–41	1.0
5 (least urgent)	746	554	74.3	39–41	14.3 (10.0–20.5)

Abbreviations: TAT = target access time, OR = odds ratio, CI = confidence interval

*Adjusted for sex, age, and registration period

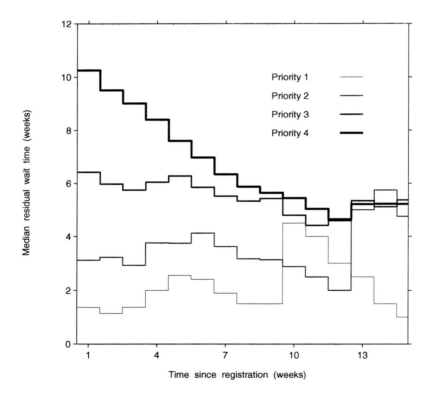

Fig. 6.2. Median residual waiting time for elective vascular surgery for a certain wait-list week, by priority group

6.2.2 Elective coronary artery bypass grafting

The objective of this study was to compare the time spent on the wait list for coronary artery bypass grafting surgery (CABG) by priority group, as described in [112] (Chapter 2). Here, we limited the analysis to patients who were registered for first-time isolated CABG. We compared the number of weeks required for specified proportions of patients to undergo the operation by priority group. The cumulative probabilities of undergoing surgery within a certain time were estimated using the product-limit method [17], as described in Chapter 3; waiting times were treated as prospective observations that were monitored from registration until the patient's last week on the list. The log-rank test, described in Chapter 3, was used to compare waiting times across priority groups [18].

The average weekly rate of surgery, that is, the total number of admissions divided by the total number of patient-weeks of follow-up, was calculated as a measure of the rate of admission within each priority group, see Chapter 3. Then, the effect size of priority group on the weekly rate of surgery was estimated by means of discrete-time survival regressions (3.87), which yield odds ratios (OR) [2], as described in Chapter 3. We used multivariable models to control for differences in age, sex, comorbidity, registration period, and hospital. Confounding variables are discussed in Chapter 4.

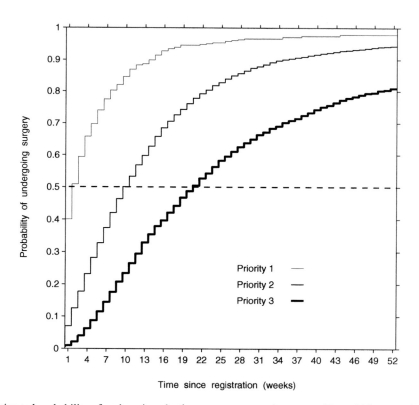

Fig. 6.3. Estimated probability of undergoing elective coronary artery bypass grafting within a certain waiting time, by priority group

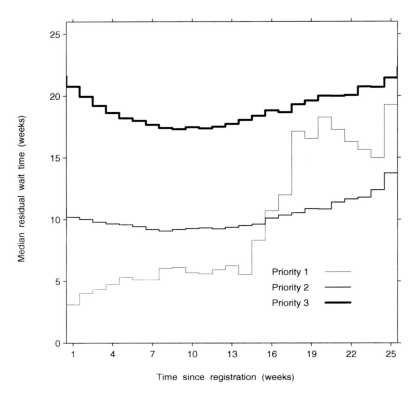

Fig. 6.4. Median residual waiting time for elective coronary artery bypass grafting for a certain wait-list week, by priority group

As expected, priority had a major influence on waiting times for CABG, with shorter times for higher-priority groups, as measured by the log-rank test (test statistic = 1414.9, df = 2, $p < 0.0001$) and the Wilcoxon test (test statistic = 1752.9, df = 2, $p < 0.0001$). Figure 6.3 shows the estimated access curves by priority group. In the nonurgent group, waiting times were such that 10%, 25%, 50%, 75%, and 80% of patients underwent surgery in 6, 11, 21, 41, and 52 weeks, respectively. In contrast, half of the patients in the semi-urgent group underwent surgery within 10 weeks, and half of those in the urgent group underwent surgery within 2 weeks. Patients had a less than 50% chance of undergoing surgery within the target access times: 40% of those in the urgent group underwent surgery within 1 week, 33% of those in the semiurgent group within 6 weeks, and 29% of those in nonurgent group within 12 weeks.

Nonurgent patients had longer median residual waiting times for all weeks since registration (Figure 6.4). Although median residual waiting times did not change drastically over time in the semiurgent and nonurgent groups, these times increased dramatically for patients in the urgent group after 15 weeks on the list. The weekly rate of surgery was greater in higher-priority groups (Table 6.3).

To evaluate the unadjusted effect of priority group on the weekly probability of admission for surgery we used a proportional odds model (equation 3.85) from discrete-time survival methods. The logit transformation of the time-dependent probability of surgery p was modeled as a linear function of priority group as defined in SAS Code B.3 (see Appendix):

$$\log\left(\frac{p_{wk}}{1 - p_{wk}}\right) = \alpha_{wk} + \beta_1\,\texttt{iurbk1} + \beta_2\,\texttt{iurbk2}\,,$$

where `iurbk1` is 1 for urgent group and 0 otherwise, `iurbk2` is 1 for semiurgent group and 0 otherwise, and `wk` indexes week on the wait list. A pooled analysis of the logistic regression models developed for each week of follow-up, treating consecutive periods of observation as ordered strata, were used to estimate common regression coefficients for the study variables.

Using SAS Code 6.2, we fit this proportional odds model. For this, we expanded the data set to create patient by week records, with an indicator variable for surgery. Then, we fitted the regression model using PROC GENMOD. By specifying `wk` as a class variable and the "noint" option in PROC GENMOD, we obtain 53 intercept estimates, $\hat{\alpha}_{wk}$, for each week on the wait list. SAS Output 6.2 shows the parameter estimates for the effect of urgent ($\hat{\beta}_1 = 1.88$, standard error $= 0.05$) and semiurgent ($\hat{\beta}_2 = 0.71$, standard error $= 0.03$) status, relative to nonurgent status. Before adjustment, the weekly odds of surgery were more than 6 times greater for patients in the urgent group and 2 times greater for those in the semiurgent group, relative to patients in the nonurgent group (Table 6.3). After adjustment (SAS code and output not shown), the weekly odds of surgery were more than 5 times greater and less than 2 times greater for patients in the urgent and semiurgent group, respectively (Table 6.3).

Therefore, we concluded that there were significant differences in access to surgery among priority groups, with larger proportions of more urgent patients undergoing CABG during every wait-list week. However, considerable variation in waiting times was observed within each priority group. Clearly, coexisting illnesses, a patient's request to postpone the operation or a surgeon's decision to ask for additional examinations before the scheduling could extend waiting times. On the other hand, cancellations because of lack of a hospital resource, such as an intensive care unit bed, could change queuing in favour of procedures that, for instance, would not require the resource.

Table 6.3. Relation between priority group and weekly rate of elective coronary artery bypass grafting, as measured by odds ratios derived from discrete-time survival regression models

Priority	No. of procedures	Total wait (patient-weeks)	Surgery rate* (95% CI)	Crude OR (95% CI)	Adjusted OR[†] (95% CI)
Urgent	570	3 056.5	18.6 (17.1–20.2)	6.58 (5.92–7.33)	5.36 (4.80–6.00)
Semiurgent	5602	86 952.5	6.4 (6.3–6.6)	2.04 (1.92–2.16)	1.59 (1.49–1.70)
Nonurgent	1406	44 595.0	3.2 (3.0–3.3)	1.00	1.00
All patients[‡]	7654	136 745.5	5.6 (5.5–5.7)	–	–

Abbreviations: OR = odds ratio from discrete survival analysis, CI = confidence interval

* Weekly surgery rate was calculated as the number of elective procedures divided by the sum of waiting times (per 100 patient-weeks)

[†] Adjusted for age, sex, registration period, comorbidity, and hospital

[‡] Includes additional patients whose priority was not available

SAS Code 6.2: Discrete-time survival regression model for effect of priority groups

```
* Create patient-week data for discrete-time survival analyses *;
data cabgex;
  set cabg;
  isx=0;
  do i=0 to wait;
    wk=i; if i=0 then wk=0.5;
    if (status=0 | status=13) & i=wait then isx=1; * indicator for surgery *;
    if wk<=52 then output; * censor at 52 weeks *;
  end;
  drop i;
run;

* Discrete-time survival model *;
proc genmod data=cabgex desc;
  where ur_bk^='U';
  class wk;
  model isx= wk iurbk1 iurbk2 /d=binomial link=logit noint;
run;
```

SAS Output 6.2: Results from discrete-time survival regression model for effect of priority groups

Analysis Of Parameter Estimates

Parameter	DF	Estimate	Standard Error	Wald 95% Confidence Limits		Chi-Square	Pr > ChiSq
Intercept	0	0.0000	0.0000	0.0000	0.0000	.	.
wk 0.5	1	-4.3058	0.0701	-4.4431	-4.1685	3777.75	<.0001
wk 1	1	-3.5705	0.0547	-3.6777	-3.4634	4263.45	<.0001
wk 2	1	-3.5536	0.0561	-3.6635	-3.4436	4012.21	<.0001
...							
wk 51	1	-4.6674	0.3817	-5.4156	-3.9192	149.49	<.0001
wk 52	1	-4.1734	0.3064	-4.7739	-3.5729	185.54	<.0001
iurbk1	1	1.8847	0.0544	1.7781	1.9913	1200.84	<.0001
iurbk2	1	0.7108	0.0307	0.6506	0.7711	535.22	<.0001
Scale	0	1.0000	0.0000	1.0000	1.0000		

6.3 Does registration period affect waiting times?

The objective of the next study was to determine whether the period of registration on a wait list affected time to isolated CABG and whether the period effect was similar across priority groups. Compared to our previous analysis in [70], we limited the analysis to patients registered for first-time isolated CABG. Using all relevant records from the provincial population-based registry of patients with coronary artery disease (CAD) identified as needing bypass surgery, as described in Chapter 2, we studied the waiting time before and after supplementary funding became available.

We compared the number of weeks from registration to surgery for equal proportions of patients in synthetic cohorts defined by five 2-year periods of registration on the wait lists: 1991–1992, 1993–1994, 1995–1996, 1997–1998, and 1999–2000. The cumulative probabilities of undergoing surgery within a certain time were estimated using the product-limit method [17], as described in Chapter 3; waiting times were treated as prospective observations that were monitored from registration until the patient's last week on the list. The log-rank test, described in Chapter 3, was used to compare waiting times across registration periods [18].

The average weekly rate of surgery, that is, the total number of admissions divided by the total number of patient-weeks of follow-up, was calculated as a measure of the rate of admission within each registration period; see Chapter 3. To measure the effect of the registration period, we used Cox regression with fixed indicator variables for registration period (3.66). The exponential of the regression coefficients for these variables gave the hazard ratios for each registration period relative to 1991–1992, a value of less than 1 indicating a lower hazard of surgery. We used multivariable models to control for differences in priority group and comorbidity. We stratified by age and sex to avoid the proportionality assumption for these variables. Confounding variables are discussed in Chapter 4.

Waiting times in 1995–1996 were such that 25%, 50%, 75%, and 90% of patients underwent surgery in 6, 15, 27, and 50 weeks, whereas half of patients in 1991–1992 and 1993–1994 underwent surgery within 9 weeks (Table 6.4).

Table 6.4. Delays in undergoing elective coronary artery bypass grafting after registration on a wait list, by registration period

Registration period	No. of patients	Procedures performed, %	Percentiles (weeks)					Maximum time
			Median (95% CI)	10th	25th	75th	90th	
1991–1992	1723	83.5	9 (9–10)	1	4	20	48	51
1993–1994	1883	84.3	9 (9–10)	2	4	19	48	52
1995–1996	1995	82.3	15 (15–16)	2	6	27	50	52
1997–1998	1884	81.6	14 (13–15)	3	7	26	44	52
1999–2000	1714	84.5	11 (10–12)	3	6	19	40	52
All periods	9199	83.2	12 (11–12)	2	5	23	46	52

Abbreviations: CI = confidence interval

The proportion of registered patients designated as having priority 1 was lowest in 1999–2000 (10.4%) and highest in 1995–1996 (36.7%), whereas the proportion designated as having priority 3 was highest was in 1999–2000 (22.3%) (Table 2.3). There was a difference in the proportion of patients undergoing surgery across registration periods, as measured by the log-rank test (test statistic = 106.1, df = 4, $p < 0.0001$). In each priority group, there was a difference in access to surgery between those registered in 1991–1992 and those registered in 1995–1996 (priority 1: test statistic = 4.1, df = 1, $p = 0.04$; priority 2: test statistic = 56.0, df = 1, $p < 0.0001$; priority 3: test statistic = 20.1, df = 1, $p < 0.0001$). For priority 1 patients, the average

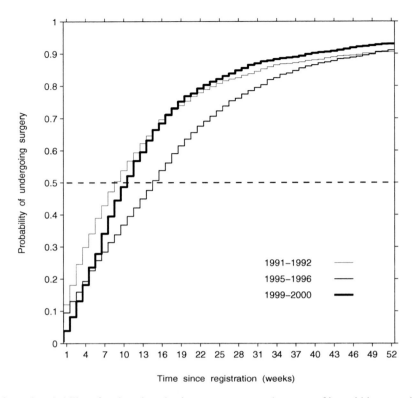

Fig. 6.5. Estimated probability of undergoing elective coronary artery bypass grafting within a certain waiting time, by registration period

weekly surgery rates declined from 36.4 per 100 patient-weeks in the 1991–1992 cohort to 17.8 in the 1995–1996 cohort and to 11.6 in the 1999–2000 cohort. For priority 2 patients, the average weekly surgery rate changed from 7.0 per 100 patient-weeks in the 1991–1992 cohort to 5.2 in the 1995–1996 cohort to 7.1 in the 1999–2000 cohort. For priority 3 patients, the average weekly surgery rate followed a similar pattern to that for priority 2 patients, with 3.7 per 100 patient-weeks in the 1991–1992 cohort, 2.6 in the 1995–1996 cohort, and 3.9 in the 1999–2000 cohort. The total number of elective and inpatient procedures increased by 13% (3681 to 4168) from 1995–1996 to 1999–2000, Tables 2.3 and 2.4. Overall, 9199 patients spent a total of 136 746 patient-weeks on the wait lists. The time to surgery increased by the middle of the decade and decreased toward the end of the decade (Figure 6.5).

To evaluate the effect of registration period on weekly surgery rate, we used a Cox regression model (equation 3.66). The hazard of surgery, $\lambda(t)$, was modeled across strata as a log-linear function of explanatory variables defined in SAS Code B.3 (see Appendix):

$$\log \lambda_s(t) = \alpha_s(t) + \beta_1 \texttt{iurbk2} + \beta_2 \texttt{iurbk3} + \beta_3 \texttt{icmc2} + \beta_4 \texttt{icmc3} + \beta_5 \texttt{icy93} + \beta_6 \texttt{icy95}$$
$$+ \beta_7 \texttt{icy97} + \beta_8 \texttt{icy99} \,,$$

where iurbk2 is 1 for semiurgent group and 0 otherwise, iurbk3 is 1 for nonurgent group and 0 otherwise, icmc2 is 1 for other comorbid conditions and 0 otherwise, icmc3 is 1 for major comorbid conditions and 0 otherwise, icy93 is 1 for 1993–1994 registration period and 0 otherwise, icy95 is 1 for 1995–1996 registration period and 0 otherwise, icy97 is 1 for 1997–1998 registration period and 0 otherwise, icy99 is 1 for 1999–2000 registration period and 0 otherwise, and $\alpha_s(t)$ is the logarithm of a baseline hazard function for stratum s defined by age group and sex. SAS Code 6.3 shows how we used PROC PHREG to fit this Cox regression model to evaluate the effect of registration period on weekly surgery rate, stratified by age and sex and adjusted for priority group and comorbidity.

Tests of the global null hypothesis (SAS Output 6.3) revealed evidence to indicate that the model explains variation in surgery rates (likelihood ratio test statistic = 1387.2, df = 8, $p < 0.0001$). The likelihood ratio test statistic (equation 3.59) is equal to the difference between -2 times the log-likelihood of the model with an intercept only and -2 times the log-likelihood of the fitted model. The -2 times the log-likelihood of the intercept only model and fitted model (see SAS Output 6.3) are 56771.9 and 55384.7, respectively. Thus, the likelihood ratio test statistic is

$$\mathrm{LRT} = 56771.9 - 55384.7 = 1387.2 \ .$$

The degrees of freedom for the chi-square distribution under the null hypothesis is equal to the number of parameters in the model, excluding the intercept, namely 8. Therefore, the p-value is the probability of observing a test statistic greater than or equal to 1387.2 from a chi-square distribution with 8 degrees of freedom, which results in a p-value less than 0.0001. SAS Output 6.3 also shows the parameter estimates for each registration period 1993–1994, 1995–1996, 1997–1998, 1999–2000 relative to 1991–1992, identified by variables icy93, icy95, icy97, and icy99.

Relative to the 1991–1992 registration period, and after adjustment for priority group at registration, comorbidity, age and sex, the conditional weekly probabilities of undergoing surgery were 30% lower among patients who were registered on a wait list in 1995–1996 (hazard ratio [HR] = 0.70, 95% CI 0.65–0.76) and 23% lower among those who were registered in 1997–1998 (HR = 0.77, 95% CI 0.71–0.83); there was no difference for those registered in 1999–2000 (HR = 0.96, 95% CI 0.89–1.03) (Table 6.5). The effect of registration period differed across priority groups (Table 6.6).

SAS Code 6.3: Cox regression model for effect of registration period

```
proc phreg data=cabg;
  where ur_bk^='U' & agecat2^=99 & sexf^='U';
  model wait05*status(1 2 3 4 5 6 7 8 9 12)= iurbk2 iurbk3 icmc2
  icmc3 icy93 icy95 icy97 icy99
    /ties=discrete;
    strata agecat2 sexf;
run;
```

SAS Output 6.3: Results from Cox regression model for effect of registration period

```
                  Model Fit Statistics

                        Without             With
        Criterion      Covariates         Covariates

        -2 LOG L       56771.907          55384.718
        AIC            56771.907          55400.718
        SBC            56771.907          55456.182


        Testing Global Null Hypothesis: BETA=0

  Test                Chi-Square       DF      Pr > ChiSq

  Likelihood Ratio     1387.1894        8        <.0001
  Score                1598.8831        8        <.0001
  Wald                 1442.4426        8        <.0001


        Analysis of Maximum Likelihood Estimates

                  Parameter    Standard
  Variable   DF   Estimate      Error    Chi-Square   Pr > ChiSq

  iurbk2      1   -1.24406     0.04914    640.8364      <.0001
  iurbk3      1   -1.95616     0.05515   1257.9714      <.0001
  icmc2       1    0.17705     0.02855     38.4495      <.0001
  icmc3       1    0.08349     0.03080      7.3462      0.0067
  icy93       1    0.02198     0.03817      0.3317      0.5647
  icy95       1   -0.35222     0.03801     85.8831      <.0001
  icy97       1   -0.26192     0.03848     46.3269      <.0001
  icy99       1   -0.04290     0.03923      1.1954      0.2742
```

Our results provide evidence that time to CABG declined after annual supplementary funding was provided to tertiary care hospitals within a single publicly funded health system. One plausible explanation is that these hospitals had the capacity to increase the number of operations. At the same time, the effect was not uniform across priority groups, which indicates that changes in clinical practice should be considered when extra funding is added to reduce wait lists.

Table 6.5. Relation between registration period and average weekly rate of elective coronary artery bypass grafting, as measured by adjusted hazard ratios derived from Cox regression models

Registration period	No. of procedures	Total wait (patient-weeks)	Surgery rate* (SE)	HR (95% CI)[†]
1991–1992	1438	23 044.5	6.2 (0.2)	1.00
1993–1994	1588	25 289.5	6.3 (0.2)	1.02 (0.95–1.10)
1995–1996	1641	34 098.0	4.8 (0.1)	0.70 (0.65–0.76)
1997–1998	1538	30 355.5	5.1 (0.1)	0.77 (0.71–0.83)
1999–2000	1449	23 958.0	6.0 (0.2)	0.96 (0.89–1.03)
All periods	7654	136 745.5	5.6 (0.1)	

Abbreviations: SE = standard error, HR = hazard ratio, CI = confidence interval

* Weekly surgery rate was calculated as the number of elective procedures divided by the sum of waiting times (per 100 patient-weeks)

[†] Adjusted for priority group and comorbidity, stratified by age and sex

Table 6.6. Access to surgery for patients registered for elective coronary artery bypass grafting, by registration period and priority group, as measured by adjusted hazard ratios* derived from Cox regression models

Registration period	Urgent Surgery rate[†] (SE)	HR (95% CI)	Semiurgent Surgery rate[†] (SE)	HR (95% CI)	Nonurgent Surgery rate[†] (SE)	HR (95% CI)
1991–1992	36.4 (3.7)	1.00	7.0 (0.2)	1.00	3.7 (0.2)	1.00
1993–1994	27.0 (2.6)	0.93 (0.67–1.29)	7.7 (0.2)	1.11 (1.02–1.21)	3.0 (0.2)	0.79 (0.66–0.94)
1995–1996	17.8 (1.2)	0.70 (0.53–0.94)	5.2 (0.2)	0.71 (0.65–0.78)	2.6 (0.2)	0.69 (0.58–0.82)
1997–1998	14.0 (1.4)	0.54 (0.39–0.75)	6.0 (0.2)	0.81 (0.75–0.89)	2.9 (0.2)	0.74 (0.62–0.88)
1999–2000	11.6 (1.5)	0.53 (0.36–0.78)	7.1 (0.2)	0.99 (0.91–1.08)	3.9 (0.2)	1.09 (0.92–1.29)

Abbreviations: SE = standard error, HR = hazard ratio, CI = confidence interval

* Adjusted for comorbidity, stratified by age and sex

[†] Weekly surgery rate was calculated as the number of elective procedures divided by the sum of waiting times (per 100 patient-weeks)

6.4 Does the type of procedure affect waiting times?

The objective of this study was to compare the time spent on the wait list for elective vascular surgery by procedure (Chapter 2). Compared to our previous analysis in [103], we added patients who were registered on the wait list after 1998.

We compared the number of weeks required for specified proportions of patients to undergo the operation by procedure. The cumulative probabilities of undergoing surgery within a certain time were estimated using the product-limit method [17], as described in Chapter 3; waiting times were treated as prospective observations that were monitored from registration until the patient's last week on the list. The log-rank test, as described in Chapter 3, was used to compare waiting times across procedures [18].

The average weekly rate of surgery, that is, the total number of admissions divided by the total number of patient-weeks of follow-up, was calculated as a measure of the rate of admission for each procedure, see Chapter 3. Then, the effect size of procedure on the weekly rate of surgery was estimated by means of the Poisson log-linear model (3.78), which yields the rate ratio (RR) [52], as described in Chapter 3.

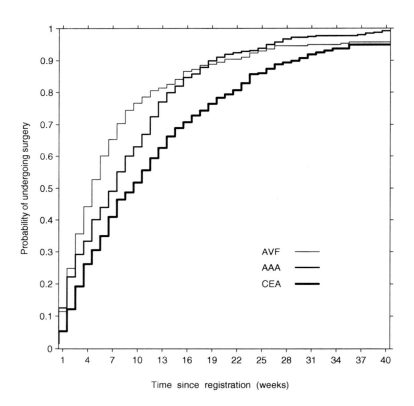

Fig. 6.6. Estimated probability of undergoing elective vascular surgery within a certain waiting time, by procedure. AVF = arteriovenous fistula, AAA = abdominal aortic aneurysm, CEA = carotid endarterectomy.

Among all patients awaiting elective surgery, there was a difference in access to surgery according to type of procedure (arteriovenous fistula (AVF), abdominal aortic aneurysm (AAA), or carotid endarterectomy (CEA)), as measured by the log-rank test (test statistic = 43.0, df = 2, $p < 0.0001$). In the AVF group, waiting times were such that 25%, 50%, 75%, and 90% of patients underwent surgery within 3, 5, 10, and 21 weeks, respectively (Figure 6.6). Waiting times were similar for the AAA group, with 50% and 90% undergoing surgery within 8 and 20 weeks, but longer for the CEA group, with 50% and 90% undergoing surgery within 10 and 30 weeks.

The weekly admission rate was lowest for patients undergoing CEA (7.4 per 100 patient-weeks) and highest for those undergoing AVF for hemodialysis (11.5 per 100 patient-weeks) (Table 6.7).

Among priority 5 patients, there was a difference in access to surgery across procedures, as measured by the log-rank test (test statistic = 98.5, df = 2, $p < 0.0001$). For these patients, waiting times to surgery were shortest for more urgent peripheral vascular disease procedures and longest for least urgent CEA procedures (Figure 6.7).

Table 6.7. Relation between type of procedure and average weekly rate of elective vascular surgery, as measured by rate ratios derived from Poisson regression models

Surgical procedure	No. of procedures	Total wait (patient-weeks)	Surgery rate* (SE)	RR (95% CI)
AAA repair	459	4389	10.5 (0.5)	0.9 (0.8–1.0)
CEA	373	5071	7.4 (0.4)	0.6 (0.6–0.7)
PVD surgery	569	5586	10.2 (0.4)	0.8 (0.7–1.0)
AVF for hemodialysis	342	2969	11.5 (0.6)	1.0

Abbreviations: SE = standard error, RR = rate ratio, CI = confidence interval,

AAA = abdominal aortic aneurysm, CEA = carotid endarterectomy,

PVD = peripheral vascular disease, AVF = arteriovenous fistula

*Weekly surgery rate was calculated as the number of procedures divided by the sum of waiting

times (per 100 patient-weeks)

Two other factors are worth discussing in this context. First, if operating room time becomes available unexpectedly, the surgeons occasionally call their wait-list managers to see if there is anyone on the list who can come in within a few hours. Therefore, partitioning a queue according to patient agreement to come at very short notice may have changed the first-come-first-served queue discipline within priority classes in favour of that procedure. Second, we hypothesize that two events, delay in scheduling operations and cancellation of booked operations, may also change waiting times.

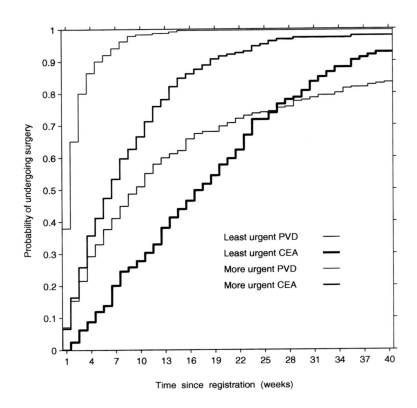

Fig. 6.7. Estimated probability of undergoing elective vascular surgery within a certain waiting time, by procedure. PVD = peripheral vascular disease, CEA = carotid endarterectomy.

6.5 Does wait-list size at registration affect time to surgery?

6.5.1 Elective vascular surgery

The objective of this study was to assess how the probability of undergoing vascular surgery within a certain period relates to the number of patients on the wait list at the time of registration [109]. We used a prospective cohort study of patients registered on the wait list for elective vascular surgery at an acute care hospital in Ontario, as briefly described in Chapter 2.

The primary outcome was time to surgery, and comparisons were made between list-size categories. List-size computation and categorization are described in Chapter 4. First, we compared the number of weeks required for specified proportions of patients to undergo the operation by list-size and batch-size categories. For each patient, the batch size of arrivals was the count of patients with higher or equal queuing priority registered on the list in the same week. The cumulative probabilities of undergoing surgery within a certain time were estimated using the product-limit method [17], as described in Chapter 3; waiting times were treated as prospective observations that were monitored from registration until the patient's last week on the list. The log-rank test, described in Chapter 3, was used to compare waiting times across list-size and batch-size categories [18].

Then, we used regression analysis of waiting times, specifically the complementary log-log model (3.92) from discrete-time survival analysis described in Chapter 3, to express the admission rate in one list-size group relative to another, with the hazard ratio being a measure of the difference between groups. Within this model, we assumed that time to surgery (in weeks) is a coarse measure and that removal from the list could occur at any time. We used multivariable models to control for differences in procedure, age, sex, and registration period. Confounding variables are discussed in Chapter 4.

For the majority of priority 1 and 2 patients, the length of the wait list at registration was 4 or fewer, whereas for the majority of priority 4 and 5 patients, it was 21 or more (Table 6.8). There was an association between list length at registration and waiting times, with shorter times for shorter lists (log-rank test statistic = 597.4, df = 2, $p < 0.0001$). When the list length exceeded 20 patients, waiting times were such that 10%, 25%, 50%, and 75% of patients underwent surgery within 3, 5, 11, and 19 weeks, respectively, whereas 50% underwent surgery within 6 weeks if 5 to 20 patients were ahead (Figure 6.8).

The batch size of arrivals in the week of registration was also associated with waiting times, with shorter times for 1 to 4 arrivals (log-rank test statistic = 38.5, df = 1, $p < 0.01$). For batch sizes of less than 5, waiting times were such that 10%, 25%, 50%, and 75% of patients underwent surgery within 1, 2, 5, and 12 weeks, respectively, whereas for batch sizes of 5 or more, 50% underwent surgery within 8 weeks. Although for patients registered on lists with fewer than 5 patients there was a difference in time to surgery for different batch sizes (log-rank test statistic = 6.7, df = 1, $p = 0.01$), there was no significant difference related to batch size for patients registered on lists with 5 to 20 patients (log-rank test statistic = 1.2, df = 1, $p = 0.27$) or more than 20 patients (log-rank test statistic = 1.5, df = 1, $p = 0.22$). Furthermore, equality of hazard ratios between batch sizes showed a difference within the smallest list-length group, as measured by the Wald test (Wald test statistic = 11.1, df = 1, $p = 0.0009$), but no difference in effect was detected within the group with batch size 5 to 20 (Wald test statistic = 2.2, df = 1, $p = 0.13$) or within the group with batch size over 20 (Wald test statistic = 1.9, df = 1, $p = 0.17$). Therefore, we report effects by batch size within the smallest list-size category only.

Table 6.8. Distribution of wait-list size and batch size for patients registered for elective vascular surgery, by priority group

Factor	All patients	Priority; no. (%) of patients				
		1	2	3	4	5
Wait-list size						
0–4	479 (25.0)	332 (96.5)	130 (87.2)	6 (2.4)	4 (1.3)	7 (0.8)
5–20	531 (27.7)	12 (3.5)	19 (12.8)	123 (49.8)	75 (24.0)	302 (35.0)
≥21	906 (47.3)	0 (0.0)	0 (0.0)	118 (47.8)	234 (74.8)	554 (64.2)
Batch size*						
1–4	1041 (54.3)	307 (89.2)	130 (87.2)	105 (42.5)	105 (33.5)	394 (45.7)
≥5	875 (45.7)	37 (10.8)	19 (12.8)	142 (57.5)	208 (66.5)	469 (54.3)

*Number of patients with higher or equal queuing priority registered on the wait list in the same week

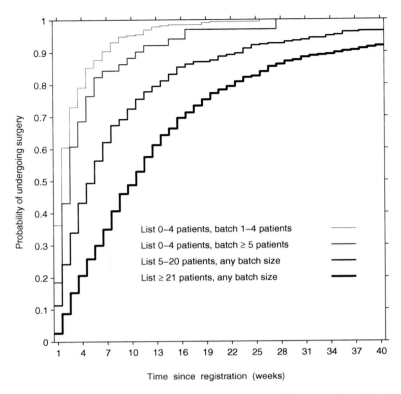

Fig. 6.8. Estimated probability of undergoing elective vascular surgery within a certain waiting time, by wait-list size and batch size

List length at registration was associated with length of wait (log-rank test statistic = 597.4, df = 2, $p < 0.0001$). To evaluate the effect of wait-list size on surgery rate we used a discrete-time survival regression model with complementary log-log link (equation 3.92). The complementary log-log transformation of the time-dependent probability of surgery p was modeled as a linear function of wait-list size and other explanatory variables as defined in SAS Code B.1 (see Appendix):

$$\log(-\log(1 - p_{\text{week}})) = \alpha_{\text{week}} + \beta_1 \texttt{wlsz2} + \beta_2 \texttt{wlsz3} + \beta_3 \texttt{ag0} + \beta_4 \texttt{ag1} + \beta_5 \texttt{ag2} + \beta_6 \texttt{sexf}$$
$$+ \beta_7 \texttt{per32} + \beta_8 \texttt{per33} + \beta_9 \texttt{proc1} + \beta_{10} \texttt{proc2} + \beta_{11} \texttt{proc3} ,$$

where `wlsz2` is 1 for list sizes 5–20 and 0 otherwise, `wlsz3` is 1 for list sizes over 21 and 0 otherwise, `ag0` is 1 for age less than 45 years and 0 otherwise, `ag1` is 1 for age between 45 and 64 years and 0 otherwise, `ag2` is 1 for age between 65 and 74 years and 0 otherwise, `sexf` is 1 for woman and 0 otherwise, `per32` is 1 for registration period 1997–1999 and 0 otherwise, `per33` is 1 for registration period 2000–2001 and 0 otherwise, `proc1` is 1 for AAA and 0 otherwise, `proc2` is 1 for CEA and 0 otherwise, `proc3` is 1 for other PVD procedures and 0 otherwise, and `week` indexes week on the wait list. The effects of explanatory variables are assumed to be constant over consecutive wait-list weeks, so we performed a pooled analysis of the regression models developed for each week of follow-up. In SAS Code 6.4, we used PROC

GENMOD to estimate the effect of wait-list size on surgery rate via a complementary log-log regression model. By specifying week as a class variable and the "noint" option in PROC GENMOD, we obtain 40 intercept estimates, $\hat{\alpha}_{week}$, for each week on the wait list. SAS Output 6.4 shows partial results of this model. Compared with the smallest list-size category, the parameter estimates for list sizes 5–20 and over 20 were $\hat{\beta}_1 = -1.19$ (SE = 0.08) and $\hat{\beta}_2 = -1.61$ (SE = 0.07), respectively. The corresponding hazard ratios from SAS Output 6.4 are shown in model 1 of Table 6.9. Patients who were registered when the list length exceeded the weekly service capacity had 70% lower conditional probability of undergoing surgery than those on a list with fewer patients (HR = 0.30, 95% CI 0.26–0.35) after adjustment for sex, age, procedure, and period. In a separate analysis, we found that registering more than 5 patients when the list was short had an independent effect (HR = 0.61, 95% CI 0.45–0.82) (see model 2 in Table 6.9).

SAS Code 6.4: Complementary log-log regression model for effect of wait-list size

```
proc genmod data=wtimesz5 desc;
  where wait>0; * exclude those with immediate access *;
  class week;
  model access=week ag0 ag1 ag2 sexf per32 per33 proc1 proc2 proc3 wlsz2 wlsz3
    /d=binomial link=cll noint;
run;
```

SAS Output 6.4: Results from complementary log-log regression model for effect of wait-list size

```
            Criteria For Assessing Goodness Of Fit

   Criterion                DF          Value        Value/DF

   Deviance                18E3       10441.1237      0.5835
   Scaled Deviance         18E3       10441.1237      0.5835
   Pearson Chi-Square      18E3       17862.6345      0.9983
   Scaled Pearson X2       18E3       17862.6345      0.9983
   Log Likelihood                     -5220.5618

Algorithm converged.

            Analysis Of Parameter Estimates

                       Standard    Wald 95% Confidence    Chi-
Parameter  DF  Estimate  Error          Limits          Square  Pr > ChiSq

wlsz2       1   -1.1943  0.0807    -1.3524   -1.0361     219.05    <.0001
wlsz3       1   -1.6102  0.0731    -1.7535   -1.4668     484.69    <.0001
```

The number of registrants on a surgical wait list affected the length of delay in providing necessary treatment. Our results suggest that a regulated list-length policy may help to reduce waiting times. Hospital

Table 6.9. Relation between wait-list size and probability of admission for elective vascular surgery in the next week, as measured by adjusted hazard ratios* derived from complementary log-log regression models

Model 1		Model 2	
Factor	**HR* (95% CI)**	**Factor**	**HR* (95% CI)**
	-	List size 0–4, batch size 1–4	1.0
List size 0–4	1.0	List size 0–4, batch size $\geq$5	0.61 (0.45–0.82)
List size 5–20	0.30 (0.26–0.35)	List size 5–20, any batch size	0.28 (0.24–0.33)
List size $\geq$21	0.20 (0.17–0.23)	List size $\geq$21, any batch size	0.18 (0.16–0.21)

Abbreviations: HR = hazard ratio, CI = confidence interval

* Adjusted for procedure, age, sex, wait-list week, and registration period

managers may also use the findings to reduce uncertainty in reporting expected waits given the current list size, which could improve resource planning.

6.5.2 Elective coronary artery bypass grafting

Previously, we determined whether the probability of undergoing CABG within a certain time was related to the number of patients on the wait list at registration in a publicly funded health system [112]. Here, we limited our analysis to patients who were registered for first-time isolated CABG. To examine the relationship between the size of a surgical wait list and the delay before undergoing treatment, we studied actual waiting times from a population-based database of patients registered for CABG surgery between 1991 and 2000 in British Columbia (Chapter 2).

For each calendar week, the list size, the number of new registrations, and the number of direct admissions immediately after angiography characterized the demand for surgery. List-size computation and categorization according to clearance times are described in Chapter 4. We compared the number of weeks required for specified proportions of patients to undergo the operation by clearance-time categories. The cumulative probabilities of undergoing surgery within a certain time were estimated using the product-limit method [17], as described in Chapter 3; waiting times were treated as prospective observations that were monitored from registration until the patient's last week on the list. The log-rank test, as described in Chapter 3, was used to compare waiting times across clearance-time categories [18]. The average weekly rate of surgery, that is, the total number of admissions divided by the total number of patient-weeks of follow-up, was calculated as a measure of the rate of admission within each group, see Chapter 3.

The effect size of clearance time on the weekly probability of admission for surgery was estimated by means of the proportional odds model (3.87) from discrete-time survival analysis, which yields the odds ratio (OR) [2], see Chapter 3. We used multivariable models to control for differences in age, sex, comorbidity, period, and hospital. Confounding variables are discussed in Chapter 4.

Table 6.10 shows the distribution of clearance times and batch sizes for patients registered for CABG, by priority group. All patients with urgent status had a clearance time of less than 1 week, whereas the clearance time was 1 month for most patients with semiurgent status (52.2%) and more than 1 month for most of those with nonurgent status (55.6%). For the majority of patients (71.9%), batch size did not exceed the weekly number of operating room slots.

The waiting times for surgery were longer for patients who were registered on lists which required longer clearance times (Table 6.11). The length of delay in undergoing treatment was associated with clearance time

Table 6.10. Distribution of clearance time and batch size for patients registered for elective coronary artery bypass grafting, by priority group

Factor	All patients	Priority; no. (%) of patients		
		Urgent	Semiurgent	Nonurgent
Clearance time				
< 1 week	1508 (16.4)	646 (100.0)	749 (11.6)	77 (3.9)
0.5 month	1273 (13.8)	0 (0.0)	999 (15.4)	253 (12.9)
1 month	3950 (42.9)	0 (0.0)	3380 (52.2)	539 (27.5)
> 1 month	2468 (26.8)	0 (0.0)	1353 (20.9)	1090 (55.6)
Batch-size*				
≤ weekly capacity	6613 (71.9)	639 (98.9)	4337 (66.9)	1541 (78.7)
> week capacity	2586 (28.1)	7 (1.1)	2144 (33.1)	418 (21.3)

*Number of patients with higher or equal queuing priority registered on the wait list in the same week

at registration, with shorter times for shorter lists (log-rank test statistic = 1103.3, $p < 0.0001$) (Figure 6.9). The average weekly surgery rate decreased with longer lists: 12.4 per 100 patient-weeks (95% CI 11.7–13.0) for group with clearance times of less than 1 week, 6.6 per 100 patient-weeks (95% CI 6.2–7.0) for group with clearance time of 0.5 month, 5.5 per 100 patient-weeks (95% CI 5.3, 5.6) for group with clearance time of 1 month, and 3.9 per 100 patient-weeks (95% CI 3.8–4.1) for group with clearance time of greater than 1 month.

To evaluate the effect of clearance time on the weekly probability of admission for surgery we used a proportional odds model (equation 3.87) from discrete-time survival methods. The logit transformation of the time-dependent probability of surgery p was modeled as a linear function of clearance time and other explanatory variables as defined in SAS Code B.3 and SAS Code B.8 (see Appendix):

$$\log\left(\frac{p_{\texttt{time}}}{1 - p_{\texttt{time}}}\right) = \alpha_{\texttt{time}} + \beta_1\texttt{age0} + \beta_2\texttt{age1} + \beta_3\texttt{age3} + \beta_4\texttt{age4} + \beta_5\texttt{sexfn} + \beta_6\texttt{icmc2} + \beta_7\texttt{icmc3}$$
$$+ \beta_8\texttt{icy93} + \beta_9\texttt{icy95} + \beta_{10}\texttt{icy97} + \beta_{11}\texttt{icy99} + \beta_{12}\texttt{ihsp2} + \beta_{13}\texttt{ihsp3} + \beta_{14}\texttt{ihsp4}$$
$$+ \beta_{15}\texttt{wlsz2} + \beta_{16}\texttt{wlsz3} + \beta_{17}\texttt{wlsz4},$$

where age0 is 1 for age less than 50 years and 0 otherwise, age1 is 1 for age between 50 and 59 years and 0 otherwise, age3 is 1 for age between 70 and 79 years and 0 otherwise, age4 is 1 for age over 80 years and 0 otherwise, sexfn is 1 for woman and 0 otherwise, icmc2 is 1 for other comorbid conditions and 0 otherwise, icmc3 is 1 for major comorbid conditions and 0 otherwise, icy93 is 1 for 1993–1994 registration period and 0 otherwise, icy95 is 1 for 1995–1996 registration period and 0 otherwise, icy97 is 1 for 1997–1998 registration period and 0 otherwise, icy99 is 1 for 1999–2000 registration period and 0 otherwise, ihsp2 is 1 for hospital 2 and 0 otherwise, ihsp3 is 1 for hospital 3 and 0 otherwise, ihsp4 is 1 for hospital 4 and 0 otherwise, wlsz2 is 1 for half month clearance time and 0 otherwise, wlsz3 is 1 for one month clearance time and 0 otherwise, wlsz4 is 1 for over one month clearance time and 0 otherwise, and time indexes week on the wait list.

A pooled analysis of the logistic regression models developed for each week of follow-up, treating consecutive periods of observation as ordered strata, were used to estimate common regression coefficients for

Table 6.11. Delays in undergoing elective coronary artery bypass grafting after registration on a wait list, by clearance time and batch size

| Factor | No. of patients | Procedures performed, % | Percentiles (weeks) | | | | | |
			Median (95% CI)	10th	25th	75th	90th	Maximum time
<1 week clearance time								
Batch size ≤ weekly capacity	1400	88.9	5 (4–5)	0	2	10	17	51
Batch size > weekly capacity	108	88.0	6 (5–8)	1	3	11	30	50
0.5 month clearance time								
Batch size ≤ weekly capacity	1046	81.1	10 (10–11)	3	6	20	39	50
Batch size > weekly capacity	227	87.7	9 (8–10)	3	6	14	17	45
1 month clearance time								
Batch size ≤ weekly capacity	2688	82.7	14 (14–15)	3	7	25	50	52
Batch size > weekly capacity	1262	88.6	10 (10–11)	2	5	19	30	52
> 1 month clearance time								
Batch size ≤ weekly capacity	1479	74.8	21 (19–22)	4	10	40	52	52
Batch size > weekly capacity	989	82.8	12 (11–14)	2	5	26	44	52

Abbreviations: CI = confidence interval

the study variables. SAS Code 6.5 shows how we used PROC GENMOD to estimate the effect of clearance time on the conditional probability of admission. Using a SAS DATA step, we created patient-week data for input into PROC GENMOD, as shown in SAS Code B.9 (see Appendix). SAS Output 6.5 shows partial results of this analysis. The ORs corresponding to SAS Output 6.5 are shown in model 1 of Table 6.12.

SAS Code 6.5: Discrete-time survival regression model for effect of clearance time

```
proc genmod data=wtimeszex desc;
   class time;
   model access=time age0 age1 age3 age4 sexfn icmc2 icmc3 icy93 icy95 icy97 icy99
       ihsp2 ihsp3 ihsp4 wlsz2 wlsz3 wlsz4
     /d=binomial link=logit noint;
run;
```

Patients registered when the list size required a clearance time of more than 1 week had 41% lower odds of undergoing surgery than those registered when list size required a clearance time of less than 1 week (OR = 0.59, 95% CI 0.54–0.65), after adjustment for age, sex, comorbidity, period, and hospital (see model 1 in Table 6.12). In a separate analysis (SAS output not shown), we found that the weekly number of new registrations exceeding weekly service capacity had an independent effect toward longer service delays when the list size at registration required a clearance time of less than 1 week (OR = 0.58, 95% CI 0.47–0.73), but not for longer lists (see model 2 in Table 6.12). By entering a continuous variable for the number of

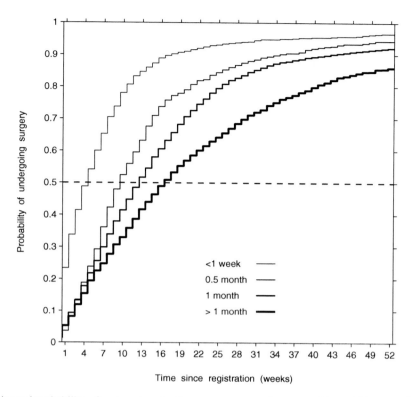

Fig. 6.9. Estimated probability of undergoing elective coronary artery bypass grafting within a certain waiting time, by clearance time

direct admissions, we found that every time an operation was performed for a patient requiring surgery without registration on a wait list, the odds of surgery for listed patients were reduced by 5% (OR = 0.95, 95% CI 0.94–0.96) (see model 3 in Table 6.12).

For wait-listed patients, we concluded that time to surgery depended on the clearance time at registration and the number of new registrations, as well as on the weekly number of patients who moved immediately from angiography to CABG without being registered on a wait list. Hospital managers may use these findings to improve resource planning and to reduce uncertainty when providing advice on expected treatment delays.

SAS Output 6.5: Results from discrete-time survival regression model for effect of clearance time

```
                Criteria For Assessing Goodness Of Fit

Criterion                    DF           Value        Value/DF

Deviance                    15E4        57467.7685       0.3943
Scaled Deviance             15E4        57467.7685       0.3943
Pearson Chi-Square          15E4       145581.0433       0.9989
Scaled Pearson X2           15E4       145581.0433       0.9989
Log Likelihood                         -28733.8842


Algorithm converged.


                    Analysis Of Parameter Estimates

                        Standard    Wald 95% Confidence     Chi-
Parameter   DF  Estimate  Error         Limits            Square  Pr > ChiSq

wlsz2        1   -0.5262  0.0453    -0.6150    -0.4374    134.94    <.0001
wlsz3        1   -0.8300  0.0373    -0.9030    -0.7569    495.71    <.0001
wlsz4        1   -1.0828  0.0425    -1.1661    -0.9995    648.96    <.0001
```

Table 6.12. Relation between both clearance time and batch size and conditional probability of elective coronary artery bypass grafting, as measured by odds ratios derived from discrete-time survival regression models

	OR* (95% CI)		
Factor	**Model 1**	**Model 2**	**Model 3**
<1 week clearance time			
Overall	1.0	–	–
Batch size ≤ weekly capacity	–	1.0	1.0
Batch size > weekly capacity	–	0.58 (0.47–0.73)	0.60 (0.48–0.74)
0.5 month clearance time	0.59 (0.54–0.65)	0.56 (0.51–0.61)	0.57 (0.52–0.62)
1 month clearance time	0.44 (0.41–0.47)	0.42 (0.39–0.45)	0.41 (0.38–0.44)
>1 month clearance time	0.34 (0.31–0.37)	0.32 (0.30–0.35)	0.31 (0.29–0.34)
Direct admissions[†]	–	–	0.95 (0.94–0.96)

Abbreviations: OR = odds ratio, CI = confidence interval

*Adjusted for age, sex, comorbidity, registration period, hospital, and wait-list week

[†] Number of additional procedures performed without wait-list registration

7

Surgery after target access time

7.1 Introduction

The length of the wait list for surgery, a common correlate of the expected wait for hospital admission, is often the only information available at the time of deciding where to seek treatment. Surprisingly little is known about how the list size at registration affects the chances of undergoing elective surgical procedures within an acceptable time. One common concern for evaluation purposes is therefore whether the proportion of late surgeries can be accurately estimated without considering the length of the wait list. Another common concern is whether the proportion of patients who undergo surgery within the target access time can be accurately estimated without considering the emergency caseload.

7.2 What proportion of patients have late surgery after registration on wait lists of different sizes?

The objective of this study was to determine the proportion of patients who underwent late coronary artery bypass grafting (CABG) after registration on wait lists of various sizes in a network of hospitals with uniform standards for timing of surgery [115]. Here, we limited our analysis to patients who were registered for first-time isolated CABG. We also examined the relation between the number of procedures performed without wait-list registration and the chances of surgery within the target access time among wait-listed patients. Using records from a population-based registry, as described in Chapter 2, we studied waiting times that had been prospectively collected for a cohort of patients registered on wait lists for CABG procedures.

In this study, the primary outcome was admission for surgery within the target access time. For procedures delayed until after the target access time, we used the number of weeks to the target time. All cases removed from wait lists without surgery and all those that exceeded target access time were treated as censored observations at 1 week after the target time. Primary comparisons were between wait-list size categories, as described in Chapter 4. The effect of list size on the weekly rate of on-time surgery was estimated by means of the proportional odds model (equation 3.87), which yields the odds ratio (OR) from discrete-time survival analysis, as described in Chapter 3, for each urgency group [2]. We used multivariable models to control for differences in patients' characteristics and significant confounders, namely age, sex, comorbidity, calendar period of registration, hospital, and the weekly number of direct admissions. These confounding variables are described in Chapter 4. For the direct admissions, we interpreted the OR as a change in the weekly odds of on-time surgery associated with one additional surgery being performed immediately after angiography.

Among those who were removed from the list before or at the target access time, 2926 (88.5%) underwent surgery, 180 (5.5%) underwent unplanned emergency admission, 62 (1.9%) continued with medical treatment, 37 (1.1%) died, 31 (0.9%) declined surgery, 22 (0.7%) were transferred to another surgeon or hospital, and 47 (1.4%) were removed for other reasons. Among those who were removed from the list after the target access time, 4728 (80.2%) eventually underwent elective surgery, 156 (2.6%) declined surgery, 134 (2.3%) underwent unplanned emergency admission, 111 (1.9%) continued with medical treatment, 76 (1.3%) were transferred to another surgeon or hospital, 54 (0.9%) died, 164 (2.8%) were removed for other reasons, and 471 (8.0%) were still on the wait list at 52 weeks.

The proportion of patients who underwent surgery within target access times varied with priority group, hospital, and clearance time (Table 7.1). For instance, the proportion who underwent surgery within target access times decreased with urgency: 39.8% of those with urgent status, 32.3% of those with semiurgent status, and 27.7% of those with nonurgent status.

Table 7.1. Characteristics of patients undergoing elective coronary artery bypass grafting within target access time, by priority group at time of registration, hospital, and clearance time for wait list

Characteristic	No. of patients	% (95% CI)
Priority at registration		
Urgent	259	39.8 (36.0–43.5)
Semiurgent	2110	32.3 (31.1–33.4)
Nonurgent	557	27.7 (25.8–29.7)
Location at registration		
Hospital 1	679	35.8 (33.7–38.0)
Hospital 2	1099	35.1 (33.4–36.8)
Hospital 3	392	18.5 (16.8–20.1)
Hospital 4	756	36.8 (34.7–38.9)
Clearance time		
< 1 week	702	46.6 (44.0–49.1)
0.5 month	428	33.6 (31.0–36.2)
1 month	1094	27.7 (26.3–29.1)
> 1 month	702	28.4 (26.7–30.2)

Abbreviations: CI = confidence interval

Over the period 1991 to 2001, two-thirds of patients were at risk of delayed surgery when registered on wait lists for isolated CABG procedures in British Columbia. Although no patients with urgent status were assigned to a wait list with clearance time exceeding 1 week, the odds of on-time surgery were reduced by 25% (OR = 0.75, 95% confidence interval [CI] 0.65–0.87) for every additional operation performed without registration on a list.

SAS Code 7.1 shows how we used PROC GENMOD to estimate the effect of wait-list size on on-time surgery for the semiurgent group. We used a DATA step to create patient-week data for on-time surgery in SAS Code B.10 (see Appendix). SAS Output 7.1 shows partial results of this analysis. With the smallest list-size category as the baseline group, the parameter estimates were −0.74 (standard error [SE] = 0.08) for a wait list with clearance time of 0.5 month, -0.83 (SE = 0.06) for a wait list with clearance time of 1 month, and -0.57 (SE = 0.07) for a wait list with clearance time of more than 1 month. The crude ORs corresponding to SAS Output 7.1 are shown in Table 7.2.

SAS Code 7.1: Discrete-time survival regression model for effect of wait-list size

```
proc genmod data=wtimeszex2 desc;
   where ur_bk2='2';
   class time;
   model access=time wlsz2 wlsz3 wlsz4 /d=binomial link=logit noint;
run;
```

SAS Output 7.1: Results from discrete-time survival regression model for effect of wait-list size

```
               Analysis Of Parameter Estimates

                        Standard  Wald 95% Confidence     Chi-
Parameter  DF  Estimate    Error        Limits          Square  Pr > ChiSq

wlsz2       1   -0.7396   0.0793   -0.8950   -0.5843      87.07    <.0001
wlsz3       1   -0.8291   0.0627   -0.9519   -0.7062     174.97    <.0001
wlsz4       1   -0.5742   0.0717   -0.7147   -0.4337      64.15    <.0001
```

Table 7.2. Relation between wait-list size and probability of elective coronary artery bypass grafting within target access time, as measured by odds ratios derived from discrete-time survival regression models

Factor	Semiurgent		Nonurgent	
	Crude OR (95% CI)	Adjusted* OR (95% CI)	Crude OR (95% CI)	Adjusted* OR (95% CI)
Clearance time				
< 1 week	1.00	1.00	1.00	1.00
0.5 month	0.48 (0.41–0.56)	0.62 (0.53–0.73)	0.86 (0.60–1.22)	0.71 (0.48–1.05)
1 month	0.44 (0.39–0.49)	0.50 (0.43–0.59)	0.37 (0.26–0.52)	0.35 (0.24–0.52)
≥1 month	0.56 (0.49–0.65)	0.46 (0.37–0.56)	0.29 (0.21–0.40)	0.28 (0.18–0.42)
Direct admission[†]	–	0.93 (0.91–0.95)	–	0.90 (0.87–0.94)

Abbreviations: OR = odds ratio, CI = confidence interval

*Adjusted for age, sex, comorbidity, registration period, hospital, and wait-list week

[†]Associated with one additional surgery performed without wait-list registration

When the wait list at registration required a clearance time of more than 1 month, patients with semi-urgent status had 54% lower odds of on-time surgery than patients registered on lists with clearance time of less than 1 week (OR = 0.46, 95% CI 0.37–0.56), after adjustment for age, sex, comorbidity, registration period, hospital, and week on the list (Table 7.2). In the nonurgent group, the odds were 72% lower (OR = 0.28, 95% CI 0.18–0.42). Every time an operation in the same hospital was performed without registration on a wait list, the odds of on-time surgery for listed patients were reduced by 7% (OR = 0.93, 95% CI 0.91–0.95) for the semiurgent group and by 10% (OR = 0.90, 95% CI 0.87–0.94) for the nonurgent group.

The chances of delayed surgery increased with wait-list size for patients needing CABG on a semiurgent or nonurgent basis. The weekly number of patients who were admitted for the operation directly from angiography, without registration on a wait list, reduced the chances of surgery within the target access time for all urgency groups. When advising patients who will be placed on a wait list about the expected time to treatment, hospital managers should take into account both the current list size and the weekly number of patients who require CABG immediately after undergoing coronary angiography.

The contribution of this study to the research on access to care is three-fold. First, it provides evidence that, for evaluation purposes, it is impossible to accurately estimate the proportion of procedures that will be delayed beyond the target access time without considering the length of the wait list. Second, it quantifies the effect of list size on the proportion of patients for whom CABG surgery will be delayed beyond target access time in a network of hospitals with uniform standards for timing of surgery. Finally, it quantifies the effect of patients undergoing the procedure without registration on a wait list on the odds of on-time surgery for patients registered on the list in that week.

7.3 What is the relation between weekly number of emergency referrals and elective admissions within the target time?

The objective of this study was to estimate the relation between the weekly number of emergency referrals and the rate of elective admissions to hospital within the target access time. To examine this relation, we used data for waiting times for elective vascular surgery and operating room records on emergency surgical procedures collected at an acute care hospital in Kingston, Ontario, as described in Chapter 2. Compared on our previous analysis in [107], we added patients who were registered on the wait list after 1999.

The primary outcomes were the number of patients who underwent surgery within the target access time and time to surgery. We used proportions to characterize the probability of a patient undergoing surgery within the target access time. As described in Chapter 3, the effects of access attributes on the odds of on-time surgery were estimated by means of logistic regressions (equation 3.57), which yielded the OR as a measure of effect size [55]. Primary comparisons were between urgency groups. Sex, age, registration period, and type of surgical procedure were entered as independent variables in the multivariable regressions to obtain adjusted effects.

The average weekly rate of on-time surgery, that is, the total number of admissions within target access times divided by the total number of patient-weeks on the list, was calculated as a measure of the rate of on-time admissions, as described in Chapter 3. To measure the effect of the weekly number of emergency referrals on the odds of elective admissions to hospital within the target access time, we estimated ORs by means of the proportional odds model (3.87) from discrete-time survival analysis, as described in Chapter 3 [2]. All cases removed from the wait list without surgery and those that exceeded the maximum target access time were treated as censored observations.

Overall, the proportion of patients who underwent surgery within the target access time was 0.47 (95% CI 0.43–0.50). The average weekly rate of surgery within the target access time was 10.2 per 100 patient-weeks (95% CI 9.6–10.8). Table 7.3 shows the relation between probabilities of undergoing vascular surgery within the target access time and the study variables. The odds of on-time surgery, derived from the logistic regression, were 28% lower in the second registration period (April 1, 1997, to March 31, 2002) (OR = 0.72, 95% CI 0.57–0.93). The odds of the procedure being done within the target access time were 34% lower for abdominal aortic aneurysm repair (OR = 0.66, 95% CI 0.38–1.15) and 43% lower for carotid endarterectomy (OR = 0.57, 95% CI 0.38–0.89) than for surgery for peripheral vascular disease.

After adjustment for the case mix and access attributes using the proportional odds model, the odds of elective admission within the target access time were, on average, 25% lower for weeks in which there were one or two emergency cases (OR = 0.75, 95% CI 0.57–0.98) and 39% lower for weeks with three or more emergency cases (OR = 0.63, 95% CI 0.48–0.84), relative to weeks with no emergency cases (Table 7.4).

In conclusion, when there was an increase in the number of emergency cases, a lower proportion of patients underwent elective surgery within the target access time. Thus, when performance of surgical services is evaluated, the probability of patients undergoing elective surgery on time should be adjusted to account for the number of emergency referrals.

Table 7.3. Relation between access factors and probability of undergoing elective vascular surgery within target access time, as measured by adjusted odds ratios derived from logistic regression

Factor	No. of procedures	Probability (95% CI)	OR* (95% CI)
Registration period			
1994–1996	295	0.48 (0.44–0.52)	1.00
1997–2002	249	0.45 (0.41–0.49)	0.72 (0.57–0.93)
Procedure			
AAA repair	105	0.32 (0.27–0.37)	0.66 (0.38–1.15)
CEA	94	0.34 (0.28–0.40)	0.57 (0.38–0.89)
PVD surgery	220	0.55 (0.50–0.60)	1.00
AVF for hemodialysis	125	0.77 (0.70–0.83)	2.95 (1.84–4.72)
Priority group			
Urgent	123	0.55 (0.48–0.61)	1.00 (0.68–1.47)
Semiurgent	143	0.30 (0.26–0.35)	0.56 (0.35–0.88)
Nonurgent	278	0.59 (0.55–0.63)	1.00

Abbreviations: OR = odds ratio, CI = confidence interval,

AAA = abdominal aortic aneurysm, CEA = carotid endarterectomy,

PVD = peripheral vascular disease, AVF = arteriovenous fistula

* Adjusted for all covariates

Table 7.4. Relation between access factors and weekly rate of elective vascular surgery within target access time, as measured by odds ratios derived from discrete-time survival regression

Factor	OR* (95% CI)
Registration period	
1994–1996	1.00
1997–2002	0.74 (0.62–0.89)
Procedure	
AAA repair	0.61 (0.38–0.99)
CEA	0.55 (0.40–0.78)
PVD surgery	1.00
AVF for hemodialysis	1.80 (1.37–2.36)
Priority group	
Urgent	8.69 (6.03–12.50)
Semiurgent	2.22 (1.45–3.41)
Nonurgent	1.00
Volume of emergency cases	
0	1.00
1 or 2	0.75 (0.56–0.98)
≥ 3	0.63 (0.48–0.84)

Abbreviations: OR = odds ratio, CI = confidence interval,

AAA = abdominal aortic aneurysm, CEA = carotid endarterectomy,

PVD = peripheral vascular disease, AVF = arteriovenous fistula

* Adjusted for all covariates

8

Adverse events while waiting

8.1 Introduction

In a patient with coronary artery disease who is to undergo coronary artery bypass grafting (CABG), delaying the operation may lead to deterioration in the patient's condition, a poor clinical outcome, an increased risk of death, or an increase in the probability of emergency admission. Recently, policy makers have called for the establishment of target access times for major operations that would minimize the risk of adverse events associated with treatment delay. Surprisingly, few studies have correlated the health effects of the presurgical wait with wait-list size at the time of registration for elective surgery. In particular, little attention has been given to the impact of delaying low-risk patients to allow treatment of those at higher risk to be expedited. The common concern is whether a patient can be referred to a specific cardiac surgeon without considering the length of the current wait list.

8.2 Do longer delays for coronary artery bypass grafting contribute to preoperative mortality among patients with less urgent need for surgery?

The objective of this study was to evaluate whether longer delays contributed to the probability of death before surgery among patients with a less urgent need for surgery using methods in Chapter 3. We prospectively studied all patients who were registered for isolated CABG in British Columbia, Canada, in 1991–2000, as described in Chapter 2. Compared on our previous analysis in [117], we limited this analysis to patients who were registered for first-time isolated CABG.

The primary outcome was the occurrence of death from any cause while awaiting CABG. To examine the relation between the length of delay and the cumulative incidence of preoperative death, we first estimated the probability of remaining on a wait list by time since registration using the product-limit method [17]. Waiting times were treated as prospective observations that were monitored from registration until the patient's last week on the list. The log-rank test was used to compare waiting times across priority groups [18]. We also estimated the time-dependent probability that a patient, who could be removed from the list as a result of surgery, death, or another competing event, dies during or before a certain wait-list week. The effect size of priority group on the weekly rate of removal was estimated by means of discrete-time survival regressions, which yielded the odds ratio (OR) [2].

We used proportions to characterize the probability that a patient would die while awaiting surgery. The effect of priority group on the odds of preoperative death was estimated by means of logistic regressions, which yielded the OR as a measure of effect size [55]. The cumulative hazard of death was estimated to investigate the accumulated risk of death over time spent on the list. The average weekly rate of death, that is, the total number of deaths divided by the total number of patient-weeks of follow-up, was calculated as a measure of the rate of death within each priority group. We then compared the rate of preoperative death per unit of waiting time across priority groups using the proportional odds model (3.87) from discrete-time survival analysis [2].

Finally, as discussed in Chapter 3, we used the cumulative incidence function (CIF) to characterize the time-dependent, marginal probability that death would occur during or before a certain wait-list week in the presence of competing wait-list events [90]. The cumulative incidence of preoperative death was compared between patients with semiurgent need for surgery and those whose need was nonurgent to isolate the effect of delaying treatment for the latter group. Matlab Code C.1 in the Appendix shows a function we used to estimate the CIF. We interpreted the cumulative incidence of preoperative death as the proportion of CABG candidates who were to undergo elective surgery but died before treatment, a number that increased over waiting time. The CIF for preoperative death is defined as the integration over time of the product of the weekly death rate and the probability of remaining on the list [21]. The CIF for death and its standard errors were estimated using nonparametric methods [90]. We used a two-sample test to compare the CIFs across priority groups [47], as described in Chapter 3.

To test for differences in the CIF between priority groups, we used competing-risk regression models based on pseudovalues of the CIF (3.96) [64]. Pseudovalues for the CIF for death were computed in the presence of surgery and other competing events at all distinct, observed event times. For each patient, the CIF pseudovalues corresponded to a series of binary variables equaling 0 before death and switched to 1 after death in the absence of censoring. We adjusted the CIF models for subject-level correlation between pseudovalues using the generalized estimation equations. The working weight matrix was fixed and estimated as a product–moment correlation matrix among the pseudovalues. We used multivariable models to control for differences in age, sex, and comorbidity. Confounding variables are discussed in Chapter 4.

Priority group was a major factor influencing the time spent on wait lists. There was a difference in the probability of remaining on the list across groups, with shorter times for greater urgency (log-rank test statistic = 1414.0, df = 2, $p < 0.0001$) (Figure 8.1). The cumulative hazard of death increased linearly with waiting times, which implied a constant hazard of death (Figure 8.2). In total, 1.0% of 9199 patients registered for CABG died on the wait list by 52 weeks: 4 (0.6%) of the 646 patients with urgent status, 54 (0.8%) of the 6481 patients with semiurgent status, and 26 (1.3%) of the 1959 patients with nonurgent status (status was unknown for 7 patients who died on the wait list). To compare the odds of preoperative death at 52 weeks between the semiurgent and nonurgent groups, we used a logistic regression model (equation 3.57). The logit transformation of the probability of preoperative death p is modeled by

$$\log\left(\frac{p}{1-p}\right) = \alpha + \beta_1 \texttt{iurbk3} ,$$

where $\texttt{iurbk3}$ is 1 for nonurgent group and 0 otherwise. SAS Code 8.1 shows how we used PROC LOGISTIC to estimate the parameters of this model, and SAS Output 8.1 shows the corresponding partial results. A test of the global null hypothesis indicated that there was marginal evidence to support that the model explains variation in the probability of death (likelihood ratio test statistic = 3.62, df = 1, $p = 0.06$). With the semiurgent group as the reference group, the parameter estimate for the nonurgent group, $\hat{\beta}_1$, was 0.47 (standard error [SE] = 0.24). Converting this parameter estimate into an OR indicates that the odds of preoperative death at 52 weeks in the nonurgent group were about 1.6 times greater than in the semiurgent group (OR = 1.6, 95% confidence interval [CI] 1.0–2.6).

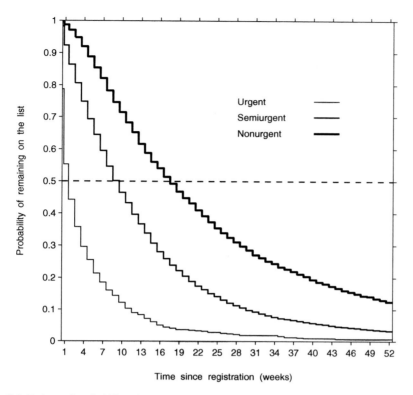

Fig. 8.1. Estimated probability of remaining on wait list, by time since registration and priority group

SAS Code 8.1: Logistic regression model for effect of priority group on preoperative death

```
proc logistic data=cabg desc;
  where ur_bk='2'|ur_bk='3';
  model death = iurbk3;
run;
```

SAS Output 8.1: Results from logistic regression model for effect of priority group on preoperative death

```
            Testing Global Null Hypothesis: BETA=0

   Test                 Chi-Square      DF      Pr > ChiSq

   Likelihood Ratio       3.6162         1        0.0572
   Score                  3.9100         1        0.0480
   Wald                   3.8405         1        0.0500


            Analysis of Maximum Likelihood Estimates

                            Standard        Wald
   Parameter    DF   Estimate    Error   Chi-Square    Pr > ChiSq

   Intercept    1    -4.7793    0.1367   1223.1644      <.0001
   iurbk3       1     0.4705    0.2401      3.8405       0.0500
```

The nonurgent group had a higher cumulative incidence of death than the semiurgent group, as measured by Gray's two-sample test (test statistic = 3.9, df = 1, $p = 0.05$) (Figure 8.3). Despite similar death rates in the semiurgent and nonurgent groups (0.62 [95% CI 0.46–0.79] and 0.58 [95% CI 0.36–0.81] per 1000 patient-weeks, respectively) (Table 8.1), patients with nonurgent status were remaining on the list longer, which contributed to higher cumulative incidence of death from any cause than in the semiurgent group (adjusted OR = 1.66, 95% CI 1.02–2.68) (Table 8.2). To estimate the effect of priority group on the cumulative incidence of death we used a CIF pseudovalue regression model (equation 3.95). The logit-transformed CIF was modeled as a linear function of priority group:

$$\text{logit}(F(\texttt{time})) = \alpha_{\texttt{time}} + \beta_1\texttt{sexfn} + \beta_2\texttt{age1} + \beta_3\texttt{age2} + \beta_4\texttt{age3} + \beta_5\texttt{age4} + \beta_6\texttt{icmc2}$$
$$+ \beta_7\texttt{icmc3} + \beta_8\texttt{iurbk3},$$

where $\texttt{sexfn}$ is 1 for woman and 0 otherwise, $\texttt{age1}$ is 1 for age less than 50 years and 0 otherwise, $\texttt{age2}$ is 1 for age between 50 and 59 years, $\texttt{age3}$ is 1 for age between 60 and 69 years, $\texttt{age4}$ is 1 for age between 70 and 79 years, $\texttt{icmc2}$ is 1 for other comorbid conditions and 0 otherwise, $\texttt{icmc3}$ is 1 for major comorbid conditions and 0 otherwise, $\texttt{iurbk3}$ is 1 for nonurgent group and 0 otherwise, and $\texttt{time}$ indexes week on the wait list. For illustration purposes, SAS Code 8.2 shows how we used PROC GENMOD to estimate the effect of priority group on the cumulative incidence of death at six time points via a CIF pseudovalue regression model. With no censoring of events, we used a DATA step to create pseudovalue data for input into PROC GENMOD (SAS Code B.11). SAS Output 8.2 shows partial results from SAS Code 8.2. With the semiurgent group as the reference group, the parameter estimate for the nonurgent group was $\hat{\beta}_8 = 0.50$ (SE = 0.24). Table 8.2 shows the corresponding ORs from parameter estimates based on the model for all time points. To estimate these ORs, we used code similar to SAS Code 8.2, but instead of 6 time points we included all 35 distinct, observed event times. The working correlation matrix had off-diagonal entries ranging from 0.19 to 0.99.

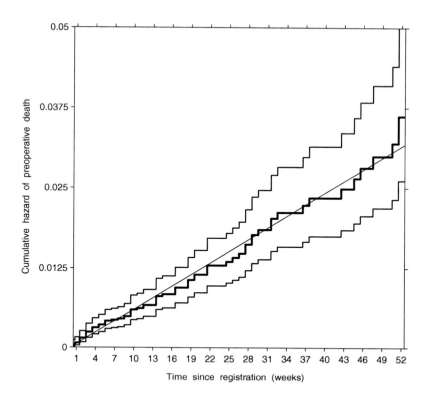

Fig. 8.2. Estimated cumulative hazard of all-cause preoperative death (and 95% confidence intervals) for semiurgent and nonurgent groups, by time since registration. The straight line is the average death rate multiplied by time.

SAS Code 8.2: Cumulative incidence function pseudovalue regression model for effect of priority group

```
proc genmod data=cabg23ex2 desc;
  where time=1|time=10|time=20|time=30|time=43|time=52;
  class ptno time;
  model psvalue = time sexfn age1 age2 age3 age4 icmc2 icmc3 iurbk3
    /dist=binomial link=logit noint;
  repeated subject=ptno
    /type=user(1 0.38652 0.32346 0.29595 0.2836 0.27266
                 0.38652 1 0.83686 0.76569 0.73373 0.70542
                 0.32346 0.83686 1 0.91495 0.87676 0.84294
                 0.29595 0.76569 0.91495 1 0.95826 0.92129
                 0.2836 0.73373 0.87676 0.95826 1 0.96142
                 0.27266 0.70542 0.84294 0.92129 0.96142 1
                 ) corrw;
run;
```

SAS Output 8.2: Results from cumulative incidence function pseudovalue regression model for effect of priority group

```
            Criteria For Assessing Goodness Of Fit

    Criterion                DF          Value      Value/DF

    Deviance                51E3       3768.3352      0.0744
    Scaled Deviance         51E3       3768.3352      0.0744
    Pearson Chi-Square      51E3      51083.1381      1.0090
    Scaled Pearson X2       51E3      51083.1381      1.0090
    Log Likelihood                    -1884.1676


                Analysis Of GEE Parameter Estimates
                Empirical Standard Error Estimates

                        Standard   95% Confidence
    Parameter   Estimate   Error       Limits          Z    Pr > |Z|

    iurbk3       0.5036    0.2453   0.0229    0.9843   2.05    0.0400
```

Table 8.1. Relation between priority group and all-cause weekly death rate for patients registered for elective coronary artery bypass grafting, as measured by odds ratios derived from discrete-time survival regression models

Priority group	No. of deaths	Total wait (patient-weeks)	Death rate[*] (95% CI)	OR[†] (95% CI)
Urgent	4	3056.5	1.31 (0.03–2.59)	2.00 (0.72–5.59)
Semiurgent	54	86952.5	0.62 (0.46–0.79)	1.00
Nonurgent	26	44595.0	0.58 (0.36–0.81)	0.94 (0.58–1.51)
All patients[‡]	91	136745.5	0.67 (0.53–0.80)	–

Abbreviations: CI = confidence interval, OR = odds ratio

[*] Per 1000 patient-weeks, calculated as the number of deaths from any causes divided by the sum of observed waiting times

[†] Adjusted for age, sex, and comorbidity

[‡] Includes additional patients for whom priority was not provided

In conclusion, the contribution of this study was twofold. First, we estimated summary probabilities that usually are not reported in prospective studies of death on wait lists. Second, we evaluated the impact of prioritizing CABG candidates on wait-list mortality. Longer delays in the nonurgent group contributed to a higher proportion of patients dying from any cause before surgery relative to the semiurgent group.

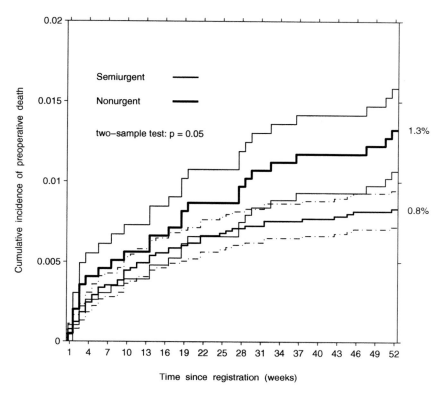

Fig. 8.3. Estimated cumulative incidence of all-cause preoperative death (and standard errors) for semiurgent and nonurgent groups, by time since registration

Table 8.2. Relation between priority group and cumulative incidence of all-cause mortality for patients registered for elective coronary artery bypass grafting, as measured by adjusted odds ratios derived from regression models for pseudovalues of cumulative incidence functions

Priority group	No. of deaths	No. of patients	% dead* (95% CI)	OR† (95% CI)
Urgent	4	646	0.6 (0.0–1.2)	–
Semiurgent	54	6481	0.8 (0.6–1.1)	1.00
Nonurgent	26	1959	1.3 (0.8–1.8)	1.66 (1.02–2.68)
All patients‡	91	9199	1.0 (0.8–1.2)	–

Abbreviations: CI = confidence interval, OR = odds ratio

* At 52 weeks

† Adjusted for age, sex, and comorbidity

‡ Includes additional patients for whom priority was not provided

8.3 What is the risk of unplanned emergency surgery among patients waiting for surgery?

8.3.1 Elective cholecystectomy

The objective of this study was to describe the distribution of times spent waiting for the operation and to assess the relation between waiting times and the risk of emergency admission [108]. We analyzed time to emergency admission for a group of 761 patients who underwent cholecystectomy after being seen in clinic for biliary colic and being placed on wait lists at two acute care centres in Ontario, from 1997 to 2000, as described in Chapter 2.

The primary outcome was emergency admission for cholecystectomy due to the worsening of symptoms while awaiting elective surgery. Cumulative probabilities of undergoing surgery electively as a function of waiting time were estimated by the product–limit method, as described in Chapter 3, with emergency cases being treated as censored observations [54, 7]. Similarly, cumulative probabilities of undergoing emergency surgery were estimated. To determine if the risk of emergency admission varied with the duration of the wait, the weekly rate, as described in Chapter 3, was calculated for the following seven intervals of time on the wait list: less than 4 weeks, 4–7 weeks, 8–11 weeks, 12–19 weeks, 20–27 weeks, 28–39 weeks, and 40–52 weeks. Because the population at risk decreases over time, the later time intervals were longer so that they would include a sufficient number of events. For each interval of waiting time, crude rate ratios (RR) were estimated relative to the first 4 weeks using the Poisson regression (3.78) [51]; see Chapter 3. Age decade, sex, calendar period of registration, and the surgeon's annual volume of cholecystectomy procedures were entered as independent variables in a multivariable regression to obtain adjusted RRs. The conditional probability of an emergency admission was estimated for the seven wait-list intervals as the number of admissions during a given interval among patients who had waited until the beginning of the interval.

Patients awaiting elective surgery spent a total of 5712 patient-weeks on wait lists. The average weekly rate of elective surgery was 12.4 (95% CI 11.5–13.3) per 100 patient-weeks. Among all patients, 25%, 50%, 75%, and 90% received access to elective surgery by 3, 6, 10, and 17 weeks, respectively (Figure 8.4).

Fifty-one patients (6.7%) had an emergency admission because of worsening symptoms while awaiting elective cholecystectomy. The average weekly rate of emergency surgery was 0.9 per 100 patient-weeks (95% CI 0.6–1.1). Among all patients, 25% and 50% underwent emergency surgery by 28 and 42 weeks, respectively (Figure 8.5).

The average weekly rate of emergency admission was 2.7 (95% CI 1.2–4.1) per 100 patient-weeks among patients who waited for 20 weeks or more and 0.9 (95% CI 0.6–1.2) per 100 patient-weeks among those who waited for less than 20 weeks. The weekly rate of emergency admission was low during the first 19 weeks on the list but increased by a factor of almost 3 after 20 weeks (RR = 2.8, 95% CI 1.9–4.1).

Although the probability of emergency admission was low during the first 19 weeks, after 20 weeks the probability started increasing and approached 40% in the interval of 40–52 weeks (Table 8.3). SAS Code 8.3 shows how we used PROC GENMOD to estimate the effect of waiting time on emergency admission via a Poisson log-linear regression model. SAS Output 8.3 shows the corresponding parameter estimates for wait-list intervals. For example, compared with the shortest interval (less than 4 weeks), the parameter estimate was −0.33 (SE = 0.40) for the interval of 4–7 weeks and 0.78 (SE = 0.51) for the interval of 20–27 weeks. The crude RRs corresponding to SAS Output 8.3 are shown in Table 8.4.

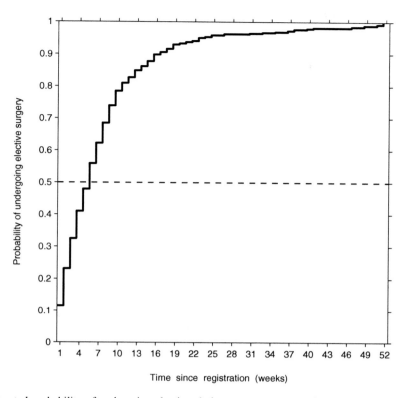

Fig. 8.4. Estimated probability of undergoing elective cholecystectomy surgery by a certain wait-list week. Reprinted from [48] with kind permission of Springer Science and Business Media.

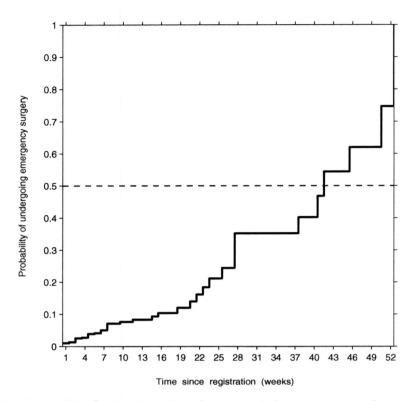

Fig. 8.5. Estimated probability of undergoing unplanned emergency cholecystectomy surgery by a certain wait-list week. Reprinted from [48] with kind permission of Springer Science and Business Media.

Table 8.3. Probability of elective and unplanned emergency admission for cholecystectomy by different periods of waiting time, conditional on remaining on the list until the start of each interval. Reprinted from [48] with kind permission of Springer Science and Business Media.

Interval (weeks)	Elective	Emergency
<4	0.32	0.02
4–7	0.44	0.02
8–11	0.49	0.03
12–19	0.53	0.03
20–27	0.43	0.11
28–39	0.33	0.19
40–52	0.60	0.40

Adjusted RRs, can be estimated with similar code, with the inclusion of confounding covariates. Relative to the first 4 weeks on the list, the rate was 1.6 times higher from 20 to 27 weeks, 2.3 times higher from 28 to 39 weeks, and 7.1 times higher from 40 to 52 weeks (Table 8.4).

SAS Code 8.3: Poisson log-linear regression model for effect of waiting time

```
proc genmod data=chole;
  model emgadm = wcat2-wcat7 /d=poisson link=log offset=ltim waldci;
run;
```

SAS Output 8.3: Results from Poisson log-linear regression model for effect of waiting time

Criteria For Assessing Goodness Of Fit

Criterion	DF	Value	Value/DF
Deviance	1733	387.5345	0.2236
Scaled Deviance	1733	387.5345	0.2236
Pearson Chi-Square	1733	3305.0896	1.9071
Scaled Pearson X2	1733	3305.0896	1.9071
Log Likelihood		-244.7672	

Analysis Of Parameter Estimates

Parameter	DF	Estimate	Standard Error	Wald 95% Confidence Limits		Chi-Square	Pr > ChiSq
Intercept	1	-4.7687	0.2425	-5.2440	-4.2933	386.59	<.0001
wcat2	1	-0.3269	0.3985	-1.1080	0.4542	0.67	0.4121
wcat3	1	0.0029	0.4491	-0.8773	0.8831	0.00	0.9949
wcat4	1	-0.4243	0.5557	-1.5135	0.6649	0.58	0.4452
wcat5	1	0.7760	0.5087	-0.2211	1.7731	2.33	0.1272
wcat6	1	0.8871	0.5557	-0.2021	1.9763	2.55	0.1104
wcat7	1	1.9065	0.5557	0.8173	2.9957	11.77	0.0006
Scale	0	1.0000	0.0000	1.0000	1.0000		

The probability that a patient on a wait list will be admitted for emergency cholecystectomy increased consistently with the duration of the wait, particularly after 20 weeks. These results have implications for developing waiting-time limits for elective surgery. The findings suggest that for patients with biliary colic who wait longer than 20 weeks for elective cholecystectomy, the risk of acute symptoms necessitating emergency surgery rises substantially.

Table 8.4. Relation between time on wait list and weekly rate of emergency admission for cholecystectomy, as measured by weekly event rates and adjusted rate ratios derived from Poisson log-linear regression models. Reprinted from *CMAJ* 2003; 169(7), Page(s) 662-665 by permission of the publisher. © Canadian Medical Association

Waiting time interval (weeks)	No. of patients at risk	Admissions/ weeks	Admission rate* (95% CI)	Crude RR[†] (95% CI)	Adjusted RR[‡] (95% CI)
< 4	761	17/2002	0.8 (0.5–1.3)	1.0	1.0
4–7	499	10/1633	0.6 (0.3–1.1)	0.7 (0.3–1.6)	0.7 (0.5–1.1)
8–11	271	7/822	0.9 (0.4–1.6)	1.0 (0.4–2.4)	1.0 (0.7–1.5)
12–19	132	4/720	0.6 (0.2–1.3)	0.7 (0.2–1.9)	0.6 (0.4–1.1)
20–27	46	5/271	1.8 (0.7–3.9)	2.2 (0.8–15.9)	1.6 (1.1–2.6)
28–39	12	4/194	2.1 (0.6–4.7)	2.4 (0.8–7.2)	2.3 (1.4–3.8)
40–52	10	4/70	5.7 (1.8–12.8)	6.7 (2.3–19.0)	7.1 (4.1–12.3)

Abbreviations: CI = confidence interval, RR = rate ratio

* Per 100 weeks of waiting time, calculated as the number of emergency admissions divided by the number of patient-weeks on the list for each interval; CIs were obtained by transforming the 95% CIs for the logarithm of observed rates

[†] Relative to the first 4 weeks

[‡] Adjusted for age decade, sex, registration period, and surgeon's annual volume of cholecystectomies

8.3.2 Elective coronary artery bypass grafting

The objectives of this study were to describe the incidence of unplanned emergency surgery among patients waiting for isolated CABG and to determine whether shorter delays reduced the probability of emergency surgery for patients with more urgent need for procedure. To estimate the time-dependent probability that a patient, who could be removed from the list through planned surgery, death, or another competing event, underwent unplanned emergency surgery during or before a certain wait-list week, we prospectively analyzed actual waiting times from a population database of all patients registered for isolated CABG between 1991 and 2000 in British Columbia, as described in Chapter 2.

The primary outcome was the occurrence of unplanned emergency admission to the participating hospital, followed by CABG, while awaiting the operation on an elective basis. Surgeons on call made the decision to operate on patients who presented to the emergency or admitting department.

To examine the relation between length of delay and cumulative incidence of emergency surgery, we first described the probability of remaining on a wait list by time since registration. This probability was estimated by the product–limit method [17], as described in Chapter 3. The log-rank test was used to compare waiting times across priority groups [18], as also described in Chapter 3.

We then compared the rate of emergency surgery per unit of waiting time across priority groups using the proportional odds model (3.87) from discrete-time survival analysis [2]; see Chapter 3. The effect size of priority group on the weekly rate of waiting outcomes was estimated by means of discrete-time survival regressions, which yielded the OR [32].

Finally, we compared the cumulative incidence of emergency surgery across priority groups using competing-risk methods. We used the CIF to characterize the time-dependent, marginal probability that unplanned emergency surgery would occur during or before a certain wait-list week in the presence of competing wait-list events [90], as described in Chapter 3. The CIF for emergency surgery and its standard errors were estimated using nonparametric methods [90]. We used a two-sample test to compare the CIFs across priority groups [47], as described in Chapter 3. To test for differences in the CIF between priority groups, we used competing-risk regression models based on pseudovalues of the CIF (3.96) [64], as described in Chapter 3 and used section 8.2. We used multivariable models to control for differences in age, sex, calendar period of registration, comorbidity, and hospital.

Overall, 314 of the 9199 CABG candidates underwent unplanned emergency surgery. By 52 weeks on the wait list, 7.7% (95% CI 5.7–9.8) of the 646 patients in the urgent group, 3.2% (2.7–3.6) of the 6481 patients in the semiurgent group, and 2.9% (2.2–3.7) of the 1959 patients in the nonurgent group had undergone emergency admission followed by CABG. The cumulative incidence of unplanned emergency surgery differed across priority groups, with higher incidence for patients with more urgent need (Gray's two-sample test statistic = 41.0, df = 2, $p < 0.0001$) (Figure 8.6). The estimated proportions of patients undergoing emergency surgery was similar for the semiurgent and non-urgent groups (adjusted OR = 0.99, 95% CI 0.71–1.39) (Table 8.5); this result was attributed to the 47% higher removal rate for patients in the semiurgent group (OR = 1.47, 95% CI 1.38–1.56), despite a higher rate of emergency surgery (0.24 [95% CI 0.20–0.27] and 0.13 [95% CI 0.09–0.16] per 100 patient-weeks, respectively) (Table 8.6).

Table 8.5. Relation between priority group and cumulative incidence of emergency admission for patients registered for elective coronary artery bypass grafting, as measured by adjusted odds ratios derived from regression models for pseudovalues of cumulative incidence functions

Priority group	No. of admissions	No. of patients	% admissions* (95% CI)	OR[†] (95% CI)
Urgent	50	646	7.7 (5.7–9.8)	2.48 (1.61–3.81)
Semiurgent	205	6481	3.2 (2.7–3.6)	0.99 (0.71–1.39)
Nonurgent	57	1959	2.9 (2.2–3.7)	1.00
All patients[‡]	314	9199	3.4 (3.0–3.8)	–

Abbreviations: CI = confidence interval, OR = odds ratio

* At 52 weeks

[†] Adjusted for age, sex, registration period, comorbidity, and hospital

[‡] Includes additional patients for whom priority was not provided

The contribution of this study was twofold. First, we estimated the summary probabilities of emergency surgery, which have not previously been reported in prospective population-based studies of preoperative outcomes for patients on surgical wait lists. Second, we found that the existing practice of queuing patients with coronary artery disease according to urgency of treatment reduced the number of emergency procedures among CABG candidates with semiurgent need. Despite a higher rate of unplanned emergency surgery in the semiurgent group than in the nonurgent group, shorter treatment delays for patients with semiurgent need resulted in similar proportions of emergency procedures over time on wait lists for both groups.

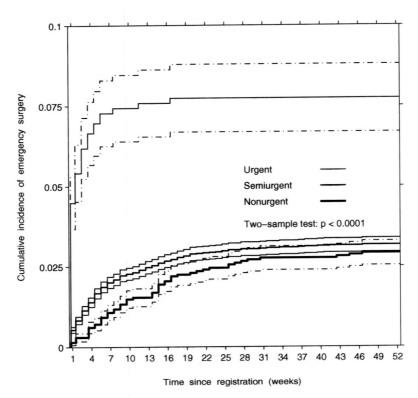

Fig. 8.6. Estimated cumulative incidence of unplanned emergency surgery (and standard error) for the three priority groups, by time since registration

Table 8.6. Relation between priority group and weekly rate of admission for unplanned emergency surgery for patients registered for elective coronary artery bypass grafting, as measured by odds ratios derived from discrete-time survival regression models

Priority group	No. of admissions	Total wait (patient-weeks)	Admission rate* (95% CI)	OR[†] (95% CI)
Urgent	50	3056.5	1.64 (1.18–2.09)	6.91 (4.54–0.52)
Semiurgent	205	86952.5	0.24 (0.20–0.27)	1.23 (0.90–1.69)
Nonurgent	57	44595.0	0.13 (0.09–0.16)	1.00
All patients[‡]	314	136745.5	0.23 (0.20–0.26)	–

Abbreviations: CI = confidence interval, OR = odds ratio

* Per 100 weeks of waiting time, calculated as the number of unplanned emergency surgeries divided by the sum of waiting times

[†] Adjusted for age, sex, registration period, comorbidity, and hospital

[‡] Includes additional patients for whom priority was not provided

8.4 What is the relation between length of the wait list at registration for coronary artery bypass grafting and chances of death while on the wait list?

The objective of this study was to compare the cumulative incidence of death while on the wait list between two groups of patients classified according to the length of the wait list at the time of their registration for CABG and to test for significant differences in the risk of death resulting from registration on a longer wait list [111]. Compared with our previous analysis in [111], the study cohort was limited to patients who were registered to undergo isolated CABG and included patients who received immediate access, as described in Chapter 2.

The primary outcome was death from any cause among patients awaiting elective CABG. The probability of remaining on the list after a certain time was estimated by the product–limit method [17], as described in Chapter 3. The log-rank test was used to compare the time to removal from the list across the study groups [18], as also described in Chapter 3.

We compared the time-dependent cumulative incidence of preoperative death before or during a certain wait-list week between two categories of wait-list size according to clearance time. List-size computations are described in Chapter 4. In this study, we categorized list size into two groups and chose 1 month clearance time as a cut-off, reasoning that registration on a wait list with a clearance time of 1 month or less would permit surgery within the target time (for semiurgent patients) of 6 weeks. We used the CIF to characterize the time-dependent probability that death would occur before or during a certain wait-list week [90], as described in Chapter 3. Using a two-sample test, as described in Chapter 3, we compared the unadjusted CIFs between urgency groups and between clearance-time categories [47].

The effect of wait-list clearance time on the weekly rate of preoperative death was estimated by means of the proportional odds model (3.87) from discrete-time survival analysis [2], as described in Chapter 3. To test for differences in the CIF, between list-size categories, we used competing-risk regression models (3.96) for the CIF with an indicator variable for a clearance time of more than 1 month [64]. The exponential of the regression coefficient for that variable gives the OR of death for clearance-time category more than 1 month relative to clearance-time category 1 month or less. For direct admissions, we interpreted the ORs as the change in the weekly odds of death while on the wait list associated with one additional surgery performed immediately after angiography. We used multivariable models to control for differences in age, sex, comorbidity, and calendar period of registration. Confounding variables are discussed in Chapter 4.

No patients with urgent status were ever registered on a wait list with a clearance time of more than 1 month. Patients with semiurgent status were registered on shorter wait lists more often than nonurgent patients (79.1% vs. 44.4%). Among those with clearance time of less than 1 month, waiting times were such that 25%, 50%, 75%, and 90% were removed from the list by 5, 10, 18, and 31 weeks, respectively (Figure 8.7), whereas among those with clearance times of more than 1 month, 50% and 90% were removed after 15 and 50 weeks, respectively. For patients with semiurgent or nonurgent status, the observed proportion of wait-list deaths by 52 weeks was lower for those patients registered on a list with clearance time of 1 month or less than for those registered on a list with clearance time of more than 1 month (0.7% [44 deaths] vs. 1.5% [36 deaths], $p < 0.005$) (Figure 8.8). After adjustment, the odds of death before surgery were 91% higher for patients on longer lists (OR = 1.91, 95% CI 1.19–3.07) (Table 8.7). The observed death rate was higher for patients registered on wait lists with clearance time of more than 1 month than for patients registered on wait lists with clearance time of 1 month or less (0.75 [95% CI 0.50–0.99] and 0.53 [95% CI 0.37-0.68] per 1000 patient-weeks, respectively; adjusted OR = 1.59 [95% CI 0.97-2.59]) (Table 8.8). Longer waiting times (log-rank test statistic = 255.3, df = 1, $p < 0.001$) and higher death rates contributed to a higher cumulative incidence of death on the wait list with a clearance time of more than 1 month (Gray's two-sample test statistic = 10.1, df = 1, $p = 0.001$).

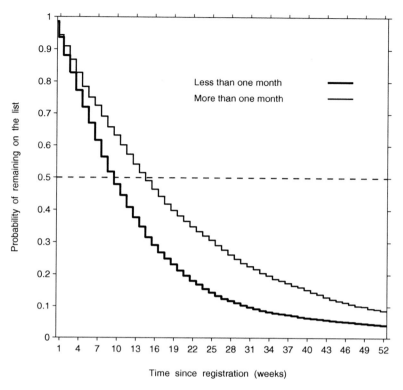

Fig. 8.7. Estimated probability of remaining on wait list for semiurgent and nonurgent priority groups, by time since registration and wait-list clearance time

The contribution of this study was twofold. First, the cumulative incidence for death on the wait list in relation to wait-list size at the time of registration for CABG has not, to our knowledge, been reported previously. After accounting for the surgery rate in semiurgent and nonurgent groups, we found that long wait lists were associated with increased probability that a patient would die before surgery. Second, physicians who advise patients to undergo revascularization with a cardiac surgeon can use these results to consider the risk of presurgical death associated with the current length of the surgeon's wait list.

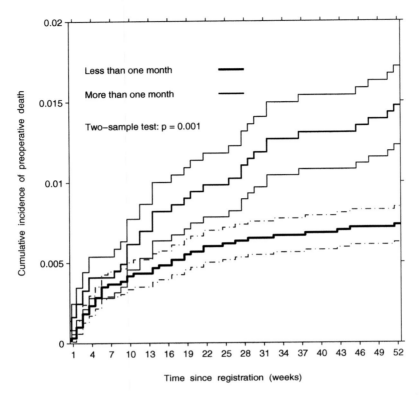

Fig. 8.8. Estimated cumulative incidence of preoperative death (and standard error) for semiurgent and nonurgent priority groups, by time since registration and wait-list clearance time

Table 8.7. Relation between wait-list clearance time and cumulative incidence of death from any cause, for semiurgent and nonurgent patients registered for elective coronary artery bypass grafting, as measured by odds ratios derived from regression models for pseudovalues of cumulative incidence functions

Factor	No. of deaths	No. of patients	% dead (95% CI)[*]	OR[†] (95% CI)
Wait-list clearance time				
< 1 month	44	5997	0.7 (0.5–0.9)	1.00
≥ 1 month	36	2443	1.5 (1.0–2.0)	1.91 (1.19–3.07)
Priority group				
Semiurgent	54	6481	0.8 (0.6–1.1)	1.00
Nonurgent	26	1959	1.3 (0.8–1.8)	1.30 (0.78–2.17)
Direct admission[‡]	–	–	–	1.00 (1.00–1.00)

Abbreviations: CI = confidence interval, OR = odds ratio

[*] At 52 weeks

[†] Adjusted for age, sex, comorbidity, registration period, and week on the list

[‡] Associated with one additional surgery performed without wait-list registration

Table 8.8. Relation between wait-list size and all-cause death rate for patients registered for elective coronary artery bypass grafting, as measured by odds ratios derived from discrete-time survival regression models

Factor	No. of deaths	Total wait (patient-weeks)	Death rate[*] (95% CI)	OR[†] (95% CI)
Wait-list clearance time				
< 1 month	44	83 378.5	0.53 (0.37–0.68)	1.00
≥ 1 month	36	48 169.0	0.75 (0.50–0.99)	1.59 (0.97–2.59)
Priority group				
Semiurgent	54	86 952.5	0.62 (0.46–0.79)	1.00
Nonurgent	26	44 595.0	0.58 (0.36–0.81)	0.73 (0.42–1.27)
Direct admission[‡]	–	–	–	1.03 (0.96–1.11)

Abbreviations: CI = confidence interval, OR = odds ratio

[*] Per 1000 weeks of waiting time, calculated as the number of deaths divided by the sum of waiting times

[†] Adjusted for age, sex, comorbidity, registration period, and week on the list

[‡] Associated with one additional surgery performed without wait-list registration

8.5 What is the relation between length of the wait list at registration for coronary artery bypass grafting and chances of unplanned emergency surgery?

In this study, we compared the cumulative incidence of unplanned emergency surgery between two groups of patients, classified according to the length of the wait list at the time of their registration for CABG and tested for significant differences in the risk of emergency surgery resulting from registration on a longer wait list [113]. We also examined the relation between the number of procedures performed without wait-list registration and the chances of unplanned emergency surgery among patients on the wait list. We used data from a prospective study of all adult British Columbia residents who were registered to undergo first-time isolated CABG, as described in Chapter 2. Compared with our previous analysis in [113], the study cohort was limited to patients who were registered to undergo isolated CABG and included patients who received immediate access, as described in Chapter 2.

The primary outcome was the occurrence of unplanned emergency surgery among patients awaiting elective CABG. Primary comparisons were between list-size categories. List-size computations are described in Chapter 4. In this study, we categorized list size into two groups, with 1 month as the dividing cut-off, reasoning that registration on a wait list with a clearance time of 1 month or less would allow the patient to undergo surgery within the target time (for semiurgent patients) of 6 weeks.

The probability of remaining on the list after a certain time was estimated by the product-limit method [17], as described in Chapter 3. The log-rank test was used to compare the time to removal from the list across the study groups [18], as described in Chapter 3. We compared the time-dependent cumulative incidence of planned surgery through unplanned emergency admission before or during a certain wait-list week between two categories of wait-list size according to clearance time. We used the CIF to characterize the time-dependent probability that unplanned emergency surgery would occur before or during a certain wait-list week [90], as described in Chapter 3. Using a two-sample test, we compared the unadjusted CIFs between urgency groups and between clearance-time categories [47], as described in Chapter 3.

The effect of wait-list clearance time on the weekly rate of unplanned emergency surgery was estimated by means of the proportional odds model (3.87) from discrete-time survival analysis [2], as described in Chapter 3. To test for differences in the CIF, between list-size categories, we used competing-risk regression models (3.96) for the CIF with an indicator variable for a clearance time of more than 1 month [64]. The exponential of the regression coefficient for that variable gives the OR of unplanned emergency surgery for patients registered on a wait list with clearance time of more than 1 month relative to those registered on a wait list with clearance time of 1 month or less. For direct admissions, we interpreted the ORs as the change in the weekly odds of unplanned emergency surgery associated with one additional surgery performed immediately after angiography. We used multivariable models to control for differences in age, sex, comorbidity, calendar period of registration, and urgency.

All patients with urgent status were registered on wait lists with clearance time of 1 month or less, and more of the patients with semiurgent status than with nonurgent status were registered on shorter wait lists (79.1% and 44.4%, respectively). After adjustment for age, sex, comorbidity, registration period, urgency, and week on the list, the rate of unplanned emergency admission was similar for patients registered on a list with clearance time of more than 1 month and those registered on a list with a clearance time of 1 month or less (OR = 1.59, 95% CI 0.97–2.59) (Table 8.9). The cumulative incidence of unplanned emergency surgery was similar between the clearance-time groups (Gray's two-sample test statistic < 0.01, df = 1, $p = 0.99$) (Figure 8.9). During 52 weeks of follow-up, an equal proportion of patients in both clearance-time categories underwent unplanned emergency surgery after registration (OR after adjustment = 1.05, 95% CI 0.79–1.40) (Table 8.10). The number of patients who underwent CABG without having been registered on a wait list in the same hospital exerted no independent effect.

Table 8.9. Relation between wait-list size and weekly rate of admission for unplanned emergency surgery for patients registered for elective coronary artery bypass grafting, as measured by odds ratios derived from discrete-time survival regression models

Factor	No. of admissions	Total wait (patient-weeks)	Admission rate* (95% CI)	OR (95% CI)[†]
Wait-list clearance time				
< 1 month	186	83 378.5	0.22 (0.19–0.26)	1.00
≥ 1 month	76	48 169.0	0.16 (0.12–0.19)	1.59 (0.97–2.59)
Priority group				
Semiurgent	205	86 952.5	0.24 (0.20–0.27)	1.00
Nonurgent	57	44 595.0	0.13 (0.09–0.16)	0.73 (0.42–1.27)
Direct admission[‡]	–	–	–	1.03 (0.96–1.11)

Abbreviations: CI = confidence interval, OR = odds ratio

* Per 100 weeks of waiting time, calculated as the number of unplanned emergency procedures divided by the sum of waiting times

[†] Adjusted for age, sex, comorbidity, registration period, and week on the list

[‡] Associated with one additional surgery performed without wait-list registration

The length of a wait list at registration had no effect on the probability that a patient with semiurgent or nonurgent status would undergo CABG through unplanned emergency admission before or during a certain wait-list week.

Table 8.10. Relation between wait-list clearance time and cumulative incidence of unplanned emergency surgery for semiurgent and nonurgent patients registered for elective coronary artery bypass grafting, as measured by adjusted odds ratios derived from regression models for pseudovalues of cumulative incidence functions

Factor	No. of admissions	No. of patients	% admissions* (95% CI)	OR[†] (95% CI)
Wait-list clearance time				
< 1 month	186	5997	3.1 (2.7–3.5)	1.00
≥ 1 month	76	2443	3.1 (2.4–3.8)	1.05 (0.79–1.40)
Priority group				
Semiurgent	205	6481	3.2 (2.7–3.6)	1.00
Nonurgent	57	1959	2.9 (2.2–3.7)	0.95 (0.69–1.29)
Direct admission[‡]	–	–	–	1.00 (1.00–1.00)

Abbreviations: CI = confidence interval, OR = odds ratio

*At 52 weeks

[†] Adjusted for age, sex, comorbidity, registration period, and week on the list

[‡] Associated with one additional surgery performed without wait-list registration

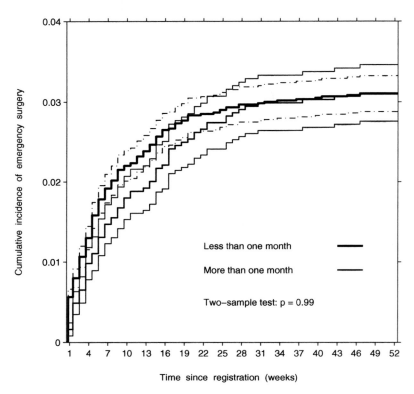

Fig. 8.9. Estimated cumulative incidence of unplanned emergency surgery (and standard errors) for semiurgent and nonurgent priority groups, by time since registration and wait-list clearance time

8.6 What is the risk of death associated with delayed surgical treatment of coronary artery disease?

The purpose of this study was to improve existing estimates of the risk of death associated with delayed surgical treatment of coronary artery disease. We estimated the time-dependent probability of death, given that CABG was not performed by certain times, using data from a prospective database of all adult patients who were accepted for isolated first-time CABG in British Columbia, as described in Chapter 2. Compared to our previous analysis in [116], here we included patients who received immediate access.

In this study, the primary outcome was the occurrence of death from any cause among patients awaiting elective CABG. We used the conditional probability function (CPF) of death to characterize the probability that a patient would die conditional on not undergoing surgery by a certain time after registration on a wait list, as described in Chapter 3. The CPF of death is based on the CIF of death and the CIF of surgery, and is defined as

$$CP_{death}(t) = \frac{F_{death}(t)}{1 - F_{surgery}(t)} .$$ (8.1)

Matlab Code C.2 in the Appendix shows a function we used to estimate the CPF. We interpreted the CPF of death as the cumulative incidence of death by a certain wait-list week among patients who had not yet undergone CABG. Using a two-sample test, we compared the unadjusted CPFs between priority groups [90]. Matlab Code C.3 in the Appendix shows a function we used to compare the CPFs.

We estimated the cumulative incidence of preoperative death, the cumulative incidence of surgery, and the probability that a patient, who may die or undergo surgery, would die if he or she did not undergo operation by certain times over the 52-week period after the decision to perform CABG. The risks were quantified separately in two groups: patients with semiurgent status at presentation were patients with either persistent unstable angina or stable angina and extensive coronary artery disease; patients with nonurgent status at presentation were stable symptomatic patients with limited disease. Among patients who had not undergone CABG by 8, 16, 32, and 52 weeks, the probabilities of death from any cause were 0.6%, 1.8%, 6.7%, and 14.5% for patients with semiurgent status and 0.6%, 1.1%, 3.4%, and 7.5% for patients with nonurgent status, respectively (Figure 8.10). For all-cause mortality, the conditional probability of death was greater in the semiurgent group than in the nonurgent group (Pepe's two-sample test statistic = 2.9, df = 1, $p = 0.002$).

The contribution of this study is the estimated conditional probabilities of death in relation to different delays in the treatment of patients requiring and suitable for CABG. These summary probabilities derived from the population-based prospective database suggest that the risk of death among those remaining untreated increases with time on a wait list. Protracted delay for revascularization carries a significant risk of death even for patients judged to be at low risk.

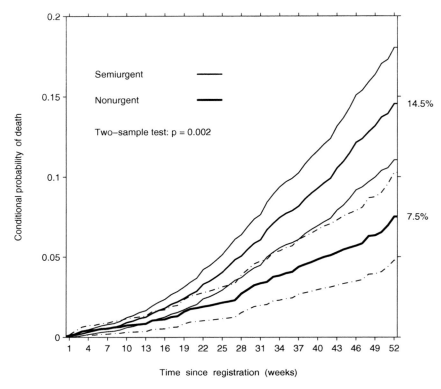

Fig. 8.10. Estimated conditional probability of preoperative death (and 95% confidence intervals) for semiurgent and nonurgent priority groups, by time since registration

9

Intermediate events

9.1 Introduction

When comparing two groups of patients, the occurrence of certain events before admission may alter the admission rate in one group, having no effect in the other; may have the same effect in both groups; or may have different effects in each group. The common concern is therefore potential bias when the groups are compared without consideration of events preceding admission. In this chapter, we first assess the effect of delays in scheduling operations on admission rates. We then assess the magnitude of the bias when access to surgery is compared between two calendar periods without data on intermediate events. This waiting-time analysis is conducted in two ways: first, using only data for the main event (elective admission) and then with additional data for the occurrence and time of an intermediate event (delay in scheduling the operation).

9.2 What is the effect of delays in scheduling an operation?

The objective of this study was to determine whether delays in scheduling an operation affected waiting time in a queue for elective vascular surgery provided by a single team of specialists. For this study, we used data from the waiting-time registry of the Division of Vascular Surgery within the Queen's University Department of Surgery, based at the Kingston General Hospital, Kingston, Ontario (Chapter 2). Compared to our previous analysis in [106], we added patients who were registered on the wait list after 1998.

A natural way to determine the impact of intermediate events, such as delay in scheduling an operation, on the outcome of interest is to use a relevant multistate model. Klein et al. have suggested using a time-dependent covariate to model (3.72) the occurrence and timing of an intermediate event that precedes the event of interest [67]. An alternative to the assumption that hazards are proportional before and after a delay, or some other time-dependent event, is to develop a model of the after-delay event hazard with a distinct baseline function for delayed patients. Notice that only patients who underwent surgery or were removed from the list after the target access times provide any information on the admission rate after delay. These observations, sometimes called late entries, must be considered left-truncated, as patients removed from the wait list without surgery before the target access time have no chance to contribute their waiting times to this analysis [22]. When data are truncated, the main impact on the analysis is that one must redefine a risk set [66]. In a left-truncated sample of n observations, in which waiting times t_i are available only for those who exceeded the target time d_i, the risk set at week j is

$$R_j = \sum_{i=1}^{n} I(d_i \leq j \leq t_i) \, ,$$

where $I(E)$ is 1 if E is true, and 0 otherwise. Andersen et al. have proposed that a separate Cox regression with late entries be used to model the rate of each possible transition in a multistate process [8]. In this study, both approaches, described in more detail in Chapter 3, were employed.

We first described the variation in times from acceptance to admission for surgery and the rates at which patients were selected from the wait list for treatment; we then estimated the effects on waiting time of different sources of delay in scheduling surgery and compared the admission rates after scheduling delays attributed to patient or hospital factors with the rate without any delay. An indicator variable is used to estimate the effect of the delay, taking on the value of 1 for those with the delay in scheduling and 0 for the rest of observations. This places the patients who received surgery after the target access times but without a scheduling delay in the reference group. Fitting the Cox model to the left-truncated data set yields partial likelihood estimates of the regression coefficients, which are interpreted as adjusted effects in the logarithmic scale.

Table 9.1. Distribution of type of scheduling delay for elective vascular surgery, by priority group

	Priority*; no (%) of patients					
	1	2	3	4	5	Total
No delay						
Within recommended time	160 (46.5)	63 (42.3)	67 (27.1)	53 (16.9)	576 (66.8)	919 (48.0)
Beyond recommended time	123 (35.8)	38 (25.5)	141 (57.1)	163 (52.1)	180 (20.9)	645 (33.7)
Delay						
Patient unfit for surgery	13 (3.8)	13 (8.7)	11 (4.5)	28 (8.9)	48 (5.6)	113 (5.9)
Patient refused	9 (2.6)	7 (4.7)	10 (4.0)	14 (4.5)	23 (2.7)	63 (3.3)
Hospital or ICU bed unavailable	23 (6.7)	19 (12.8)	6 (2.4)	43 (13.7)	4 (0.5)	95 (5.0)
Operating room unavailable	12 (3.5)	5 (3.4)	7 (2.8)	5 (1.6)	8 (0.9)	37 (1.9)
Doctor's decision	4 (1.2)	4 (2.7)	5 (2.0)	7 (2.2)	23 (2.7)	43 (2.2)
Total	344	149	247	313	862[†]	1915

Abbreviation: ICU = intensive care unit

* Adjusted for age, sex, calendar period of registration, comorbidity, and hospital

[†] One patient with unknown reason for delay

For most (81.7%) of the patients there was no delay (Table 9.1). Scheduling delays were most frequent for patients with priority 2 status (32.2% of patients) and least frequent for those with priority 5 status (12.3%) (Table 9.1). The proportion of patients waiting beyond target access times ranged from 20.9% of patients with priority 5 status to 57.1% of those with priority 3 status. Admissions with a scheduling delay tended to have longer waiting times (Table 9.2). Patients without a scheduling delay had the highest probability of undergoing surgery for all weeks on the list, whereas those with a scheduling delay had the lowest probability of undergoing surgery (Figure 9.1).

Table 9.2. Characteristics of waiting-time distributions for elective vascular surgery, by priority group and type of admission

	No. of patients	No. (%) censored	Median no. of weeks of waiting (95% CI)
Admission with no delay in scheduling			
Priority			
1 (most urgent)	344	72 (20.9)	2 (1–2)
2	149	54 (36.2)	3 (3–4)
3	247	47 (19.0)	7 (6–8)
4	313	103 (32.9)	10 (8,–2)
5 (least urgent)	863	167 (19.4)	18 (16–21)
Overall	1916	443 (23.1)	6 (6–7)
Admission with a delay in scheduling			
Priority			
1 (most urgent)	61	4 (6.6)	3 (3–4)
2	48	1 (2.1)	7 (5–9)
3	39	7 (17.9)	9 (7–14)
4	97	13 (13.4)	12 (12–14)
5 (least urgent)	107	57 (53.3)	35 (30–41*)
Overall	352	82 (23.3)	13 (12–15)
Admission beyond recommended time, with no delay in scheduling			
Priority			
1 (most urgent)	123	9 (7.3)	3 (3–4)
2	38	1 (2.6)	5 (4–6)
3	141	7 (5.0)	10 (8–11)
4	163	4 (2.5)	12 (10–13)
5 (least urgent)	180	38 (21.1)	24 (22–26)
Overall	645	59 (9.1)	12 (11–13)

*Data derived from all waiting-time observations by censoring any
delayed patient at their delay time

Among those who had surgery, only 50.9% underwent the operation within target access times. This proportion varied significantly across priority group, from 17.4% of patients with priority 4 status to 74.3% of patients with priority 5 status. Patients with any delay in scheduling surgery had longer waiting times than patients without delays (Figure 9.1). Using all observations, we modeled the time-dependent effect of a delay. Then using a left-truncated sample of waiting times that exceed target access times, we modeled the effect of a delay.

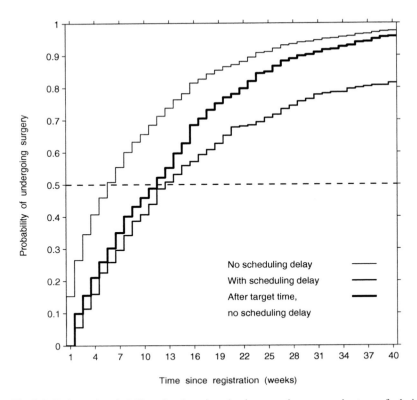

Fig. 9.1. Estimated probability of undergoing elective vascular surgery, by type of admission

In the first analysis, the time-dependent effect of delay on the hazard of admission was modeled using Cox regression (3.71). The hazard of admission, $\lambda(t)$, was modeled across strata as a log-linear function of explanatory variables defined in SAS Code B.1 (see Appendix):

$$\log \lambda_s(t) = \alpha_s(t) + \beta_1 \texttt{pr1} + \beta_2 \texttt{pr2} + \beta_3 \texttt{pr3} + \beta_4 \texttt{pr4} + \beta_5 \texttt{sexf} + \beta_6 \texttt{ag0} + \beta_7 \texttt{ag1} + \beta_8 \texttt{ag2} + \beta_9 \texttt{idelay} \,,$$

where $\texttt{pr1}$ is 1 for priority group 1 and 0 otherwise, $\texttt{pr2}$ is 1 for priority group 2 and 0 otherwise, $\texttt{pr3}$ is 1 for priority group 3 and 0 otherwise, $\texttt{pr4}$ is 1 for priority group 4 and 0 otherwise, $\texttt{sexf}$ is 1 for woman and 0 otherwise, $\texttt{ag0}$ is 1 for age less than 45 years and 0 otherwise, $\texttt{ag1}$ is 1 for age between 45 and 64 years and 0 otherwise, $\texttt{ag2}$ is 1 for age between 65 and 74 years and 0 otherwise, $\texttt{idelay}$ is 1 if scheduling delay and t is greater than target access time and 0 otherwise, and $\alpha_s(t)$ is the logarithm of a baseline hazard function for stratum s defined by registration period. SAS Code 9.1 shows how we used PROC PHREG to estimate this regression model with a time-dependent effect of a scheduling delay. SAS Output 9.1 shows the partial results of this analysis. A test of the global null hypothesis indicated that there was evidence to support that the model explains variation in the hazard of admission (likelihood ratio test statistic = 590.4, df = 9, $p < 0.0001$). The parameter estimate for the time-dependent effect of a delay was $\hat{\beta}_9 = -0.67$ (standard error [SE] = 0.08). The adjusted HR corresponding to SAS Output 9.1 is shown in Table 9.3. According to the first analysis, the admission rate was 49% lower (hazard ratio [HR] = 0.51, 95% confidence interval [CI] 0.44–0.60) for those with a delay than for those without a delay. Using the likelihood ratio test, we compared the models before and after adjustment for scheduling delay:

$$LRT = 9293.0 - 9214.4 = 78.6 .$$

Based on a chi-square distribution with 1 degree of freedom, a test statistic of 78.6 indicates strong evidence to support that scheduling delays explained the variation in the hazard of admission for surgery.

In the second analysis, we used a similar Cox regression model to study the effect of scheduling delay, but the time at risk was left-truncated at the target access time. SAS Code 9.2 shows how we used PROC PHREG to estimate this regression model with an effect for scheduling delay. SAS Output 9.2 shows the partial results of this analysis. A test of the global null hypothesis indicated that there was evidence to support that the model explains variation in the hazard of admission (likelihood ratio test statistic = 177.2, df = 9, $p < 0.0001$). The HR value of 0.55, derived from the left-truncated sample in the second analysis, also suggested that the admission rate for patients with scheduling delays was about half the rate for patients who waited longer than the target access time but without any delays.

In a separate analysis, we studied the impact of different sources of delay using all observations. For certain sources of delay, the admission rate was 20% to 70% lower than the rate for admissions without a delay, independent of the urgency of the surgical intervention (see model 1 in Table 9.4). The admission rate for patients with scheduling delays due to reasons other than operating room unavailability was 51% lower than the rate for patients admitted without the delays. However, there were no differences between the admission rate for patients delayed because the operating room was unavailable and the rate for patients admitted without the delays (see model 2 in Table 9.4).

The contribution of this study was twofold. First, we developed a method to infer how intermediate events, occurring randomly between registration and admission, affect waiting time. Second, these results provide evidence that delays in scheduling operations lengthen waiting times independent of the patients' urgency status. These findings support the concern expressed by Lewis et al. [71] and others that waiting time for elective surgery is not simply determined by how many patients are on the wait list or by how urgently they need treatment, but also by wait-list management practices.

SAS Code 9.1: Cox regression model for time-dependent effect of scheduling delay

```
proc phreg data=vasc;
  where wait>0;
  model wait*status(1 2 3 4 5 6 7 8)= pr1 pr2 pr3 pr4
    sexf ag0 ag1 ag2 idelay /ties=exact risklimits;
    idelay=del;
    if wait<gl then do; idelay=0; end;
  strata fy;
run;
```

SAS Output 9.1: Results from Cox regression model for time-dependent effect of scheduling delay

```
        Testing  Global  Null  Hypothesis:  BETA=0

 Test                    Chi-Square      DF       Pr > ChiSq

 Likelihood Ratio          590.3995       9        <.0001
 Score                     814.7548       9        <.0001
 Wald                      685.9355       9        <.0001


         Analysis  of  Maximum  Likelihood  Estimates

              Parameter    Standard
 Variable   DF   Estimate     Error   Chi-Square   Pr > ChiSq

 idelay      1   -0.66536    0.07860    71.6511      <.0001

         Analysis  of  Maximum  Likelihood  Estimates

                    Hazard    95% Hazard Ratio
           Variable  Ratio    Confidence Limits

           idelay    0.514     0.441      0.600
```

Table 9.3. Relation between priority group and admission for elective vascular surgery before and after adjustment for scheduling delays, as measured by hazard ratios derived from Cox regression models

	HR (95% CI)			
	For all observations		For left-truncated sample	
	Before adjustment	After adjustment[*]	Before adjustment	After adjustment[*]
Priority				
1 (most urgent)	6.02 (5.14–7.05)	7.77 (6.57–9.19)	7.12 (4.86–0.43)	8.66 (5.88–2.78)
2	2.51 (2.07–3.05)	3.36 (2.73–4.18)	3.54 (2.49–5.03)	4.53 (3.16, 6.48)
3	1.38 (1.18–.61)	1.51 (1.29–1.77)	2.24 (1.69–2.98)	2.33 (1.75–3.11)
4	1.00 (0.87–1.15)	1.17 (1.01–1.36)	1.76 (1.36–2.29)	2.03 (1.55, 2.64)
5 (least urgent)	1.0	1.0	1.0	1.0
Scheduling delay				
No	–	1.0	–	1.0
Yes	–	0.51 (0.44–0.60)	–	0.55 (0.46–0.65)
−2 log likelihood	9293.0	9214.4	4100.6	4051.5

Abbreviations: HR = hazard ratio, CI = confidence interval

[*] Adjusted for sex and age and stratified on the registration period

SAS Code 9.2: Cox regression model for effect of scheduling delay

```
proc phreg data=vasc;
  where outcome>1;
  model (gl,wait)*status(1 2 3 4 5 6 7 8) = pr1 pr2 pr3 pr4
    sexf ag0 ag1 ag2 del /ties=exact risklimits;
  strata fy;
run;
```

SAS Output 9.2: Results from Cox regression model for effect of scheduling delay

Testing Global Null Hypothesis: BETA=0

Test	Chi-Square	DF	Pr > ChiSq
Likelihood Ratio	177.2392	9	<.0001
Score	187.5150	9	<.0001
Wald	178.2214	9	<.0001

Analysis of Maximum Likelihood Estimates

Variable	DF	Parameter Estimate	Standard Error	Chi-Square	Pr > ChiSq
del	1	-0.60630	0.08912	46.2810	<.0001

Analysis of Maximum Likelihood Estimates

Variable	Hazard Ratio	95% Hazard Ratio Confidence Limits	
del	0.545	0.458	0.649

Table 9.4. Relation between both priority group and specific reason for scheduling delay and admission for elective vascular surgery among patients who waited longer than target times, as measured by hazard ratios derived from Cox regression models

	HR* (95% CI)	
	Model 1	**Model 2**
Priority		
1 (most urgent)	8.82 (5.96–13.07)	8.83 (5.98–13.05)
2	4.74 (3.30–6.80)	4.69 (3.27–6.71)
3	2.50 (1.87–3.34)	2.37 (1.78–3.15)
4	2.03 (1.55–2.65)	2.08 (1.59–2.71)
5 (least urgent)	1.00	1.00
Reason for scheduling delay		
No delay	1.00	1.00
OR unavailable	1.22 (0.85–1.74)	1.16 (0.81–1.66)
Patient unfit	0.38 (0.28–0.52)	–
Patient refused	0.44 (0.32–0.59)	–
Hospital or ICU bed unavailable	0.83 (0.64–1.08)	–
Doctor's decision	0.30 (0.19–0.48)	–
Other than OR unavailable	–	0.49 (0.41–0.59)

Abbreviations: HR = hazard ratio, CI = confidence interval,

OR = operating room, ICU = intensive care unit

*Adjusted for sex and age and stratified on the calendar year

9.3 What is the effect of registration period in the presence of delays?

Previously, we determined the effect of excluding data related to delays in scheduling operations in calculating the difference in admission rates between two registration periods [105]. Compared to our previous analysis, we added patients who were registered on the wait list after 1999. Data were taken from a waiting-time registry that was set up to prospectively collect data for a cohort of patients accepted for elective vascular surgery in the Department of Surgery, Queen's University, Kingston, Ontario, as described in Chapter 2.

The cumulative probability of admission as a function of time spent on the wait list was estimated by the product-limit method [54], as described Chapter 3. All cases removed from the wait list without surgery were treated as censored observations [7]. By using the log-rank and Wilcoxon tests, we were able to compare the likelihood of admission by registration period [65].

The target access time, measured in weeks, was used as a proxy for the delay in scheduling surgery. To measure the effect of scheduling delays, we used Cox regression with a time-dependent indicator variable that changed from 0 to 1 at the time of the delay (3.72) [67], as described in Chapter 3. The exponential of the regression coefficient for this variable gave the HR for delayed patients relative to those who were not delayed, a value of less than 1 indicating a lower hazard resulting from delay. First, the registration period effect was estimated without taking intermediate events into account. Second, the occurrence and timing of delays in scheduling operation were entered into the analysis. Lastly, the occurrence and timing of scheduling delays for each registration period were accounted for. The estimates were derived from the Cox regression model with three time-dependent indicator variables coded in such a way that the before-delay admission rate in the first registration period (July 1, 1994 to March 31, 1997) was the reference.

We used multivariable models to control for differences in patient characteristics and significant confounders. In particular, we entered indicator variables for sex and urgency status. When performing the Cox regression analysis, we stratified by surgical procedure and age group to avoid the proportionality assumption for these variables.

There was no association between waiting times and registration period (log-rank test statistic = 3.6, df = 1, $p = 0.06$) (Figure 9.2). The average weekly rate of surgery was 10.5 per 100 patient-weeks (95% CI 9.6–11.4) in the first registration period (July 1, 1994 to March 31, 1997) and 9.3 per 100-patient weeks (95% CI 8.8–9.9) in the second registration period (April 1, 1997 to March 31, 2002). Median time to surgery was similar in the two registration periods (6 weeks [95% CI 5–6] for the first registration period and 7 weeks [95% CI 6–7] in the second registration period). After a delay, the average weekly surgery rate remained higher for patients enrolled during the first registration period (9.2 per 100 patient-weeks, 95% CI 6.6–11.8) than for patients enrolled during the second registration period (6.7 per 100 patient-weeks, 95% CI 5.8–7.5).

In the first analysis, the effect of registration period on the hazard of admission, $\lambda(t)$, was modeled across strata as a log-linear function of explanatory variables (model 1):

$$\log \lambda_s(t) = \alpha_s(t) + \beta_1 \text{pr1} + \beta_2 \text{pr2} + \beta_3 \text{pr3} + \beta_4 \text{pr4} + \beta_5 \text{sexf} + \beta_6 \text{per2} ,$$

where pr1 is 1 for priority group 1 and 0 otherwise, pr2 is 1 for priority group 2 and 0 otherwise, pr3 is 1 for priority group 3 and 0 otherwise, pr4 is 1 for priority group 4 and 0 otherwise, sexf is 1 for woman and 0 otherwise, per2 is 1 for the second registration period and 0 otherwise (see SAS Code B.1 in Appendix), and $\alpha_s(t)$ is the logarithm of a baseline hazard function for stratum s defined by age group and type of surgery. Without adjustment for scheduling delays, the admission rate for the second registration period was 23% lower than for the first registration period (see model 1 in Table 9.5). In the next analysis, we adjusted for scheduling delays using model 2:

$$\log \lambda_s(t) = \alpha_s(t) + \beta_1 \text{pr1} + \beta_2 \text{pr2} + \beta_3 \text{pr3} + \beta_4 \text{pr4} + \beta_5 \text{sexf} + \beta_6 \text{per2} + \beta_7 \text{idelay} ,$$

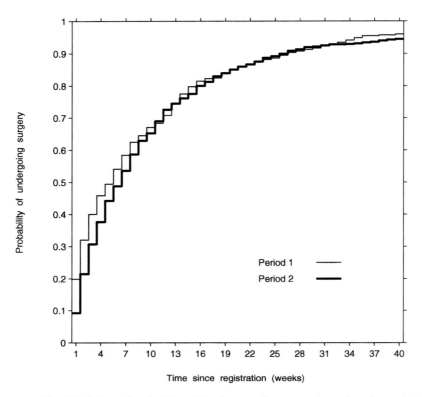

Fig. 9.2. Estimated probability of elective vascular surgery, by registration period

where `idelay` is 1 if scheduling delay and t exceeds target access time and 0 otherwise. The difference between the registration periods remained significant after adjustment for scheduling delays (see model 2 in

Table 9.5. Relative rates of admission without (model 1) and with (models 2 and 3) adjustment for scheduling delays

	RR* (95% CI)		
Factor	**Model 1**	**Model 2**	**Model 3**
1994–1996	1.0	1.0	1.0
After delay	–	–	0.59 (0.43–0.80)
1997–2002	0.77 (0.69–0.86)	0.82 (0.73–0.91)	0.85 (0.73–0.99)
After delay	–	–	0.57 (0.48–0.67)
Delay	–	0.58 (0.50–0.67)	–

Abbreviations: RR = relative rate, CI = confidence interval

*Adjusted for sex, age, urgency, and type of surgery

Table 9.5). However, the difference between registration periods was minimal for comparisons of admission rates before any delay occurred (see model 3 in Table 9.5). In the last analysis, we adjusted for scheduling delays for each registration period (model 3):

$$\log \lambda_s(t) = \alpha_s(t) + \beta_1 \mathtt{pr1} + \beta_2 \mathtt{pr2} + \beta_3 \mathtt{pr3} + \beta_4 \mathtt{pr4} + \beta_5 \mathtt{sexf} + \beta_6 \mathtt{iadelayper1} + \beta_7 \mathtt{ibdelayper2}$$
$$+ \beta_8 \mathtt{iadelayper2},$$

where `iadelayper1` is 1 if scheduling delay and t exceeds target access time in period 1 and 0 otherwise, `ibdelayper2` is 1 if scheduling delay and t is within target access time in period 2 and 0 otherwise, and `iadelayper2` is 1 if scheduling delay and t exceeds target access time in period 2 and 0 otherwise. For patients with a scheduling delay, the admission rate among those enrolled in the first and second registration periods was 41% and 43% lower, respectively, than among those enrolled in the first registration period without any scheduling delays (see model 3, after delay, in Table 9.5).

These results provide evidence that patients experiencing a delay in the scheduling of an operation have a lower admission rate after the event causing the delay. Thus, potential for bias exists when a between-group comparison of waiting time is done without adjustment for an intermediate event that may occur before elective admission.

10

Survival benefit of coronary artery bypass grafting

10.1 Introduction

Randomized trials and observational studies have demonstrated the survival benefits conferred by coronary artery bypass grafting (CABG). In practice, however, personal reasons, scheduling procedures, or surgical wait lists can delay CABG after decision to operate has been made. Hence, any treatment-related effect found in such studies does not include additional potential benefit for patients who died before they could undergo the scheduled procedure. Hannan and colleagues argued that estimates of survival benefits from undergoing CABG should account for the total number of deaths, including those that resulted from a longer wait for required revascularization [50]. The analysis presented in this chapter, which concludes that undergoing CABG rather than remaining untreated reduces the risk of death by half, is more relevant to patients perspective because it compares the long-term prognosis for both alternatives: if CABG is performed or if the patient remains untreated. In our view, such estimates introduce a methodological innovation, whereby deaths among untreated patients are used to estimate the death rate for the treated group if they had remained untreated.

10.2 What is the survival benefit of coronary artery bypass grafting?

The objective of this study was to compare survival after the treatment decision between patients who underwent CABG and those who remained untreated. We used observational data from a population-based registry of patients with established coronary artery disease for whom surgical revascularization was indicated and planned, as described in Chapter 2.

The primary outcome was death from any cause after the decision for surgery was made. The time to death was counted as the number of months from the decision to treat (or the last request for an operating room) until death or 5 years after the treatment decision or December 31, 2002, whichever came first. We also studied deaths that occurred after surgery but during the same hospital admission [20] and deaths that occurred after discharge from the hospital. The time to death for patients who underwent surgery and were alive at discharge was counted as the number of months from discharge to death or 5 years after discharge or December 31, 2002, whichever came first. We excluded an additional 70 records from the analysis of long-term postoperative survival because the discharge date was invalid or missing.

We measured the effect of surgical revascularization on survival after the treatment decision in two cohorts of patients, namely semiurgent and nonurgent, categorized by symptoms, coronary anatomy, and left ventricular function. To measure the treatment-related effect, we used Cox regression with a time-dependent indicator variable that changed from 0 to 1 after surgery (3.72) [42], as described in Chapter 3. The exponential of the regression coefficient for this variable gave the hazard ratio (HR) for treated patients relative to those who remained untreated, a value of less than 1 indicating a lower hazard resulting from having undergone CABG.

We also studied whether survival differed significantly among patients who waited for CABG longer than the target access time (6 weeks for patients in the semiurgent group and 12 weeks for those in the nonurgent group [70]), using a separate model with two time-dependent indicator variables for CABG performed before and after the target access time. To test for differences in postoperative survival between patients who underwent CABG within and after the target access time, we used Cox regression with fixed covariates [31]. The timing of surgery was an indicator variable, a value of 1 denoting CABG within the target access time. Point estimates and confidence intervals (CIs) for HRs were calculated for each urgency group and for the combined cohorts.

We used multivariable models to control for differences in patient characteristics and significant confounders (summarized in Table 10.1). In particular, we entered two indicator variables, one for coexisting medical conditions (congestive heart failure, diabetes mellitus, chronic obstructive pulmonary disease, rheumatoid arthritis, or cancer [83]) and other coexisting chronic conditions, as defined by Romano et al [97]. Presentation without coexisting conditions was the reference category. When performing the Cox regression analysis, we stratified by age and sex to avoid the proportionality assumption for these variables. To assess whether the estimated models were consistent with our data, we used the likelihood ratio test.

Of patients in the semiurgent group, 32.2% underwent elective CABG within the target access time, 55.2% underwent the procedure after the target access time, and 3.2% underwent the procedure via unplanned emergency admission (Table 10.1). Among those in the nonurgent group, 28.3% underwent elective CABG within the target access time, 48.1% underwent the procedure beyond the target access time, and 3.1% underwent the procedure via unplanned emergency admission (Table 10.1). About 10% of patients died during the first 5 years after the treatment decision: 80 died while awaiting surgery, 141 after withdrawal from the wait list, 100 postoperatively during the admission for CABG, and 563 after hospital discharge (Table 10.2).

The effect of surgery on the hazard of death, $\lambda(t)$, was modeled across strata using a log-linear function of explanatory variables (3.66):

$$\log \lambda_s(t) = \alpha_s(t) + \beta_1 \text{icmc2} + \beta_2 \text{icmc3} + \beta_3 \text{icy} + \beta_4 \text{ihsp2} + \beta_5 \text{ihsp3} + \beta_6 \text{ihsp4} + \beta_7 \text{iurbk2}$$
$$+ \beta_8 \text{isx} ,$$

where icmc2 is 1 for other comorbid conditions and 0 otherwise, icmc3 is 1 for major comorbid conditions and 0 otherwise, icy is 1 for 1997–2000 registration period and 0 otherwise, ihsp2 is 1 for hospital 2 and 0 otherwise, ihsp3 is 1 for hospital 3 and 0 otherwise, ihsp4 is 1 for hospital 4 and 0 otherwise, iurbk2 is 1 for semiurgent group and 0 otherwise, isx is 1 if received admission to surgery by t and 0 otherwise, and $\alpha_s(t)$ is the logarithm of a baseline hazard function for stratum s defined by age group and sex. SAS Code 10.1 shows how we used PROC PHREG to fit this time-dependent effect for surgery via a Cox regression model.

SAS Output 10.1 shows the partial results of this analysis. A test of the global null hypothesis indicated that there was evidence to support that the model explains variation in the hazard of death (likelihood ratio test statistic = 123.4, df = 8, $p < 0.0001$). The estimated regression coefficient for the time-dependent effect for surgery is -0.57 (standard error [SE] = 0.09). Among those who underwent CABG, the hazard of death was 57% of that in the untreated group (adjusted HR = 0.57, 95% CI 0.48–0.68) (Table 10.3).

SAS Code 10.1: Cox regression model for time-dependent effect of surgery

```
proc phreg data=cabg;
 where ur_bk='2'|ur_bk='3';
 model twlsdthcm*dthstssc(98 99)=icmc2 icmc3 icy ihsp2 ihsp3 ihsp4 iurbk2 isx
  /ties=breslow rl;
  strata sexfn agecat2;
  if (status5y=0|status5y=12|status5y=13) & twlsdthcm>=waitm0 then isx=1; else isx=0;
run;
```

SAS Output 10.1: Results from Cox regression model for time-dependent effect of surgery

```
          Testing Global Null Hypothesis: BETA=0

  Test                  Chi-Square      DF      Pr > ChiSq

  Likelihood Ratio       123.3951        8        <.0001
  Score                  135.3492        8        <.0001
  Wald                   131.9699        8        <.0001


         Analysis of Maximum Likelihood Estimates

              Parameter    Standard
  Variable  DF  Estimate      Error   Chi-Square  Pr > ChiSq

  isx        1   -0.56603    0.09103    38.6599      <.0001
```

The effect was stronger when CABG was performed within the target access time: adjusted HRs were 0.51 (95% CI 0.42–0.63) for early treatment and 0.70 (95% 0.58–0.84) for late treatment (Wald chi-square for the difference between hazard ratios = 12.8, df = 1, $p < 0.01$) (Table 10.3).

Compared with untreated patients, the hazard of death was 40% lower for patients in the semiurgent group who underwent the procedure (adjusted HR = 0.60, 95% CI 0.49–0.75) and 52% lower for patients in the nonurgent group who underwent the procedure (adjusted HR = 0.48, 95% CI 0.34–0.67) (Table 10.4).

Of the 7431 patients who underwent CABG, 100 (1.3%) died postoperatively during the same hospital admission. The odds of in-hospital death among patients who underwent CABG was 37% lower for those who underwent CABG within the target access time than beyond (adjusted HR = 0.63, 95% CI 0.41–0.98) (Table 10.5).

Of the 7261 patients who underwent CABG and survived surgery, 563 (7.8%) died within 5 years. Among these patients, the hazard of death for those who underwent CABG within target access time relative to those who underwent the procedure beyond the target access time was 21% lower for patients in the semiurgent group (adjusted HR = 0.79, 95% CI 0.65–0.96) and 19% lower for those in the nonurgent group (adjusted HR = 0.81, 95% CI 0.52–1.25) (Table 10.5).

In conclusion, our estimates that account for patients who died before they could undergo a required CABG indicate a significant survival benefit of performing early surgical revascularization. In particular, we found a significant mortality reduction for patients registered to undergo coronary revascularization on the non-urgent basis. The survival benefit of CABG was greater when patients underwent the operation within the target time, suggesting that some of the benefit was lost by the delay beyond the target time.

Table 10.1. Characteristics of patients registered for elective coronary artery bypass grafting, by type of access to surgery

Characteristic	All patients (n=8440)	Unplanned emergency (n=266)	Within target time (n=2643)	After target time (n=4522)	Remained untreated (n=1009)
Age group (years)					
<50	8.1	2.8	31.3	54.1	11.8
50–59	22.0	3.0	28.8	56.7	11.5
60–69	38.1	3.2	31.6	53.6	11.6
70–79	29.8	3.3	32.9	51.9	11.9
≥80	1.9	2.4	31.7	41.5	24.4
Sex					
Women	17.7	4.1	30.9	51.5	13.4
Men	82.3	2.9	31.4	54.0	11.6
Priority group					
Semiurgent	76.8	3.2	32.2	55.2	9.4
Nonurgent	23.2	3.1	28.3	48.1	20.5
Comorbidity					
Major conditions[†]	21.5	3.7	33.3	49.4	13.6
Other conditions[‡]	25.9	3.6	35.9	48.8	11.7
None	52.6	2.7	28.2	57.6	11.4
Coronary anatomy					
Left main	11.9	2.6	40.5	48.7	8.2
Multivessel[§]	80.2	3.1	30.0	54.9	12.0
Limited[‖]	7.9	4.0	31.2	47.1	17.6
Registration Period					
1991–1992	18.4	3.2	40.2	44.9	11.8
1993–1994	20.9	2.9	38.3	47.2	11.6
1995–1996	20.5	3.1	21.6	62.9	12.5
1997–1998	20.8	3.7	25.3	58.2	12.8
1999–2000	19.4	2.9	32.1	54.0	11.0
Location of registration					
Hospital 1	20.8	3.7	35.8	46.2	14.3
Hospital 2	33.6	2.6	35.4	51.9	10.1
Hospital 3	24.2	2.8	18.6	60.2	18.4
Hospital 4	21.4	3.8	34.9	56.0	5.3

*For the column with data for all patients, the percentages within each characteristic are calculated with reference to the total number of patients (that is, percentages sum to 100 within each characteristic). For the columns with data according to access to surgery, the percentages are calculated with reference to the number of patients within each category (that is, percentages sum to 100 across rows)

[†]Congestive heart failure, diabetes mellitus, chronic obstructive pulmonary disease, rheumatoid arthritis, or cancer

[‡]Peripheral vascular disease, cerebrovascular disease, dementia, peptic ulcer disease, hemiplegia, renal disease, or liver disease

[§]Three- or two-vessel disease with stenosis of the proximal left anterior descending artery

[‖]Two-vessel disease with no lesion in the proximal left anterior descending artery or one-vessel disease with stenosis of the proximal left anterior descending artery

Table 10.2. Characteristics of patients registered for elective coronary artery bypass grafting who died during follow-up

Characteristic	Time of death*; % of patients[†]			
	On wait list (n=80)	After withdrawal (n=141)[‡]	During admission (n=100)	After discharge (n=563)[§]
Age group (years)				
<50	6.3	3.5	2.0	2.7
50–59	21.3	14.2	17.0	13.5
60–69	36.3	27.0	36.0	34.8
70–79	35.0	45.4	43.0	44.8
≥80	1.3	9.9	2.0	4.3
Sex				
Women	8.8	24.8	26.0	17.1
Men	91.3	75.2	74.0	82.9
Priority group				
Semiurgent	67.5	68.1	88.0	82.4
Nonurgent	32.5	31.9	12.0	17.6
Comorbidity				
Major conditions[‖]	32.5	37.6	34.0	32.5
Other conditions**	25.0	25.5	24.0	24.0
None	42.5	36.9	42.0	43.5
Coronary anatomy				
Left main	7.5	9.2	12.0	13.5
Multivessel[††]	82.5	79.4	84.0	81.3
Limited[‡‡]	10.0	11.3	4.0	5.2
Registration Period				
1991–1992	16.3	15.6	28.0	26.1
1993–1994	28.8	19.1	14.0	20.2
1995–1996	22.5	27.7	23.0	24.3
1997–1998	21.3	23.4	21.0	20.6
1999–2000	11.3	14.2	14.0	8.7
Location of registration				
Hospital 1	13.8	32.6	9.0	19.4
Hospital 2	32.5	27.0	52.0	34.1
Hospital 3	43.8	30.5	15.0	21.5
Hospital 4	10.0	9.9	24.0	25.0

*On wait list = any preoperative death while on the wait list for surgery;

after withdrawal = any preoperative death after removal from the wait list without surgery;

during admission = any death after surgery during the same hospital admission;

after discharge = any death after hospital discharge

[†] The percentages within each characteristic (as listed in column 1) are calculated with reference to the number of patients within each category at time of death

[‡] Within 5 years of registration date

[§] Within 5 years of hospital separation date, excluding two patients with unknown separation date

[‖] Congestive heart failure, diabetes mellitus, chronic obstructive pulmonary disease, rheumatoid arthritis, or cancer

**Peripheral vascular disease, cerebrovascular disease, dementia, peptic ulcer disease, hemiplegia, renal disease, or liver disease

[††] Three- or two-vessel disease with stenosis of the proximal left anterior descending artery

[‡‡] Two-vessel disease with no lesion in the proximal left anterior descending artery or one-vessel disease with stenosis of the proximal left anterior descending artery

Table 10.3. Hazard ratios for death at any time after registration for coronary artery bypass grafting, comparing treated and untreated patients and comparing surgery within and after target access times, derived from Cox regression models

Time-dependent treatment effect*	Deaths/patients	HR (95 % CI)	
		Unadjusted	Adjusted[†]
Model 1 (Treatment indicator)			
Treated vs untreated	624/7431 vs 221/1009	0.60 (0.50–0.71)	0.57 (0.48–0.68)
Model 2 (Treatment indicator by target time)			
Early surgery vs untreated	218/2794 vs 221/1009	0.53 (0.44–0.65)	0.51 (0.42–0.63)[‡]
Late surgery vs untreated	406/4637 vs 221/1009	0.68 (0.57–0.82)	0.70 (0.58–0.84)[‡]
Model 3 (Treatment indicator by target time and admission type)			
Early surgery vs untreated	205/2643 vs 221/1009	0.53 (0.43–0.65)	0.51 (0.41–0.62)[§]
Late surgery vs untreated	394/4522 vs 221/1009	0.68 (0.57–0.81)	0.70 (0.58–0.84)[§]
Unplanned emergency vs untreated	25/266 vs 221/1009	0.68 (0.45–1.04	0.68 (0.44–1.03)

Abbreviations: HR = hazard ratio, CI = confidence interval

* Among 8440 patients who were to undergo the operation

[†] Adjusted for comorbidity, registration period, hospital and priority group, and stratified by age and sex

[‡] Significant difference between regression estimates (Wald chi-square = 12.8, df = 1, $p < 0.01$)

[§] Significant difference between regression estimates (Wald chi-square = 12.9, df = 1, $p < 0.01$)

Table 10.4. Hazard ratios for death at any time after registration for coronary artery bypass surgery, comparing treated and untreated patients, derived from Cox regression models

	HR (95 % CI)	
Time-dependent treatment effect[*]	**Semiurgent group**	**Nonurgent group**
Overall survival (time-dependent treatment effect, as no. of deaths/no. of patients)[†]		
Deaths/patients:		
Treated patients	526/5874	98/1557
Untreated patients	150/607	71/402
Model 1 (treatment indicator)		
Treated vs untreated		
Unadjusted hazard ratio	0.61 (0.49–0.75)	0.46 (0.33–0.63)
Adjusted hazard ratio[‡]	0.60 (0.49–0.75)	0.48 (0.34–0.67)
Model 2 (treatment indicator by target time)		
Early surgery vs untreated		
Unadjusted hazard ratio	0.56 (0.44–0.70)	0.38 (0.24–0.59)
Adjusted hazard ratio[‡]	0.56 (0.44–0.70)	0.38 (0.24–0.59)
Late surgery vs untreated		
Unadjusted hazard ratio	0.70 (0.56–0.87)	0.53 (0.37–0.76)
Adjusted hazard ratio[‡]	0.75 (0.60–0.93)	0.57 (0.40–0.83)
Model 3 (treatment indicator by target time and admission type)		
Early surgery vs untreated		
Unadjusted hazard ratio	0.56 (0.44–0.71)	0.35 (0.22–0.55)
Adjusted hazard ratio[‡]	0.56 (0.44–0.71)	0.35 (0.22–0.56)
Late surgery vs untreated		
Unadjusted hazard ratio	0.70 (0.56–0.87)	0.52 (0.36–0.74)
Adjusted hazard ratio[‡]	0.75 (0.60–0.93)	0.56 (0.39–0.81)
Unplanned emergency vs untreated		
Unadjusted hazard ratio	0.58 (0.35–0.96)	0.99 (0.47–2.07)
Adjusted hazard ratio[‡]	0.61 (0.37–1.02)	0.88 (0.41–1.86)

Abbreviations: HR = hazard ratio, CI = confidence interval

[*] Unless indicated otherwise

[†] Among 8440 patients who registered to undergo the operation

[‡] Adjusted for comorbidity, registration period, hospital and priority group, and stratified by age and sex

Table 10.5. Odds ratios for in-hospital death, derived from logistic regression models, and hazard ratios for postoperative death, derived from Cox regression models

Outcome	All patients	Semiurgent group	Nonurgent group
In-hospital* (deaths/admissions)			
Early surgery	30/2794	–	–
Late surgery	70/4637	–	–
Unadjusted OR (95 % CI)	0.71 (0.46–1.09)	–	–
Adjusted OR (95 % CI)†	0.63 (0.41–0.98)	–	–
Long-term postoperative survival‡ (no. of deaths/total follow-up years)			
Early surgery	–	163/9505	31/2390
Late surgery	–	300/15 171	67/4008
Unadjusted HR (95 % CI)	–	0.86 (0.71–1.04)	0.79 (0.52–1.21)
Adjusted HR (95 % CI)§	–	0.79 (0.65–0.96)	0.81 (0.52–1.25)

Abbreviations: OR = odds ratio, CI = confidence interval, HR = hazard ratio

* Among 7431 patients who were admitted for surgery

† Adjusted for age, sex, comorbidity, registration period, hospital, and priority group

‡ Within 5 years from discharge date among 7261 patients who underwent surgery and did not die in hospital, after removal of 70 patients with invalid discharge dates

§ Adjusted for comorbidity, registration period, hospital, priority group and mode of admission, and stratified by age and sex

Part III

Appendices

A

Data dictionaries

A.1 Data dictionary for coronary artery bypass grafting inpatients

Table A.1. Data dictionary for records of inpatients admitted for coronary artery bypass grafting

Variable	Description	Source	Code
BCCR_ID	Patient identifier	BCCR	\<Text\>
AGECAT	Age decade	BCCR	0 – < 20 years
			1 – 20–29 years
			2 – 30–39 years
			. . .
			8 – ≥90 years
SEXF	Sex	BCCR	0 – Man
			1 – Woman
UR_SX	Urgency at surgery	BCCR	0 – Emergency
			1 – Urgent
			2 – Semiurgent
			3 – Nonurgent
			U – Unknown
CM_CH	Comorbidities from Charlson index	Hospital Separations	0, 1, 2, 3, or 4 (≥ 4)
CM_SX	Major comorbidities	Hospital Separations	1 – CHF, diabetes, COPD, rheumatism or cancer
			0 – Other
INST_SX	Location at surgery	BCCR	Hospital 1, 2, 3, or 4

| SX_DATE | Operation date | BCCR | mm/dd/yyyy |

Abbreviations: BCCR = British Columbia Cardiac Registry, CHF = congestive heart failure, COPD = chronic obstructive pulmonary disease

A.2 Data dictionary for vascular

Table A.2. Data dictionary for records of patients awaiting elective vascular surgery

Variable	Description	Code
CR	Patient identifier	Positive integer
SEX	Sex	Male – Man
		Female – Woman
AGE	Age (years)	Positive integer
SX_DX	Diagnosis	1 – Repair of AAA more 8 cm
		2 – Repair of AAA 6 to 8 cm
		3 – Repair of AAA 5 to 6 cm
		4 – CEA for symptomatic disease
		5 – CEA for asymptomatic disease
		6 – Bypass surgery for PVD with pain at rest
		7 – Other PVD surgeries
WL_DATE	Wait-list registration date	mm/dd/yyyy
ADM_DATE	Wait-list removal date	mm/dd/yyyy
ADM_WIT	Admission within target access time	Yes – Within target access time
		No – Beyond target access time
		N/A – Removed without surgery
		WL – Still on wait list
IF_NOT	Reason for delay	0 – No delay
		1 – Patient unfit for surgery
		2 – At patient request
		3 – No hospital bed
		4 – No intensive care unit bed
		5 – Operating room unavailable
		6 – Doctor's decision
		7 – Length of wait list
TAKEN_OF	Reason for removal	0 – Received surgery
		1 – Still on wait list
		2 – Cancellation of booked surgery due to patient condition
		3 – Patient condition prevented booking surgery

		4 – Health deterioration: stroke, rupture, TIA
		5 – Death
		6 – Patient refused to undergo booked surgery
		7 – Patient improved
		8 – Patient decided against surgery
EXPR1	Indicator of AVF procedure	1 – AVF
		0 – Otherwise
EXPR2	Indicator of ABF procedure	1 – ABF
		0 – Otherwise
EXPR3	Indicator of other bypass surgery	1 – Other bypass surgery
		0 – Otherwise
EXPR4	Indicator of VV or ligation,	1 – VV or ligation if no AVF
		0 – Otherwise

Abbreviations: AAA = abdominal aortic aneurysm, CEA = carotid endarterectomy,

PVD = peripheral vascular disease, AVF = arteriovenous fistula,

ABF = aorto-bifemoral bypass, VV = varicose veins, TIA = transient ischemic attack

A.3 Data dictionary for cholecystectomy

Table A.3. Data dictionary for records of patients awaiting elective cholecystectomy

Variable	Description	Code
AG_CA1	Age decade	1 – <25 years
		2 – 25–34 years
		3 – 35–44 years
		4 – 45–54 years
		5 – 55–64 years
		6 – 65–74 years
		7 – ≥75 years
SEXF	Sex	0 – Man
		1 – Woman
EP	Registration period	1 – 1997–1998
		2 – 1998–1999
		3 – 1999–2000
VT	Surgeon's annual case volume	1 – <20
		2 – 20–40
		3 – >40
EVENT	Surgery type	1 – Elective surgery
		2 – Emergency surgery
WAIT	Waiting time from registration to surgery	Integer for number of weeks

B

SAS code

B.1 DATA steps

B.1.1 Preparing data set on access to vascular surgery

SAS Code B.1: DATA step to create analytical data set

```
/*********************************************************
 * Program: \vascular\sas\common\step_1.sas
 *
 * Input data: "booklib" is a library that contains
 * the data set, "vasc1", of original records
 *
 * Description: to apply exclusion criteria,
 * create categorical and indicator variables,
 * and compute waiting times
 *********************************************************/

data vasc2;
  set booklib.vasc1;
  **********************
  * Exclusion criteria *
  **********************;
  if age < 25 then delete;

  *****************
  * Priority group *
  *****************;
  /* AAA > 8 cm or PVD with pain */
  if sx_dx =1 or sx_dx =6 then urgstat=1;
  /* AAA 6-8 cm */
  if sx_dx =2 then urgstat=2;
  /* AAA 5-6 cm */
  if sx_dx =3 then urgstat=4;
  /* CEA symptomatic */
  if sx_dx =4 then urgstat=3;
```

```
/* CEA asymptomatic, other PVD, ABF, other bypass surgery, VV */
if sx_dx =5 or sx_dx =7 then urgstat=5;
/* indicator variables and target access times */
pr1=0; pr2=0; pr3=0; pr4=0; pr5=0;
if urgstat=1 then do; pr1=1; gl=1; end;
if urgstat=2 then do; pr2=1; gl=2; end;
if urgstat=3 then do; pr3=1; gl=3; end;
if urgstat=4 then do; pr4=1; gl=4; end;
if urgstat=5 then do; pr5=1; gl=13; end;


****************
* Age category *
****************;
if age^=. then do;
  age_cat=99; ag0=0; ag1=0; ag2=0; ag3=0;
  if age<45 then do; age_cat=0; ag0=1; end;
  if 45<=age<65 then do; age_cat=1; ag1=1; end;
  if 65<=age<75 then do; age_cat=2; ag2=1; end;
  if 75<=age then do; age_cat=3; ag3=1; end;
end;


***********************
* Registration period *
***********************;
m=month(wl_date); d=day(wl_date); yo=year(wl_date);
if mdy(06,1,1994)> mdy(m,d,yo) then delete;
if mdy(06,01,1994)<= mdy(m,d,yo) <=mdy(03,31,1995) then do; fy=1; end;
if mdy(04,01,1995)<= mdy(m,d,yo) <=mdy(03,31,1996) then do; fy=2; end;
if mdy(04,01,1996)<= mdy(m,d,yo) <=mdy(03,31,1997) then do; fy=3; end;
if mdy(04,01,1997)<= mdy(m,d,yo) <=mdy(03,31,1998) then do; fy=4; end;
if mdy(04,01,1998)<= mdy(m,d,yo) <=mdy(03,31,1999) then do; fy=5; end;
if mdy(04,01,1999)<= mdy(m,d,yo) <=mdy(03,31,2000) then do; fy=6; end;
if mdy(04,01,2000)<= mdy(m,d,yo) <=mdy(03,31,2001) then do; fy=7; end;
if mdy(04,01,2001)<= mdy(m,d,yo) <=mdy(03,31,2002) then do; fy=8; end;
* 2 period categories ;
per1=0; if fy<4 then per1=1;
per2=1-per1;
* 3 period categories ;
per3=0; per31=0; per32=0; per33=0;
if fy<4 then do; per3=1; per31=1; end; * 94/95 to 96/97 ;
if fy>=4 & fy<7 then do; per3=2; per32=1; end; * 97/98 to 99/00 ;
if fy>=7 then do; per3=3; per33=1; end; * 00/01 to 01/02 ;


*******
* Sex *
*******;
if sex^="" then do; sexf=0; if sex='Female' then sexf=1; end;
```

```
*************
* Procedure *
*************;
/* Surgical procedures, sx_dx is original codes
sx_dx sx
1 1 - Repair of AAA more 8 cm
2 2 - Repair of AAA 6 to 8 cm
3 3 - Repair of AAA 5 to 6 cm
4 4 - CEA for symptomatic disease
5 5 - CEA for asymptomatic disease
6 6 - Bypass surgery for PVD with pain at rest
7 7 - Other PVD surgeries
      8 - AVF for hemodialysis access
      9 - Aorto-bifemoral bypass
     10 - Other bypass surgeries
     11 - VV or veins ligation
*/
sx=sx_dx;
if expr1=1 then sx=8; * AVF ;
if expr3=1 and sx_dx=7 then sx=10; * other bypass surgeries for PVD ;
if expr2=1 then sx=9; * ABF - aorto-bifemoral bypass ;
   if expr4=1 and expr1^=1 then sx=11; * VV or ligation ;
proc=1; * AAA ;
if sx_dx =6 and sx =9 then sx=6;
if sx=4 or sx=5 then proc=2; * CEA ;
if sx=6 or sx=9 or sx=10 then proc=3; * PVB ;
if sx=7 or sx=11 then proc=3; * other PVD surgeries ;
if sx=8 then proc=4; * AVF ;
/* indicator variables */
proc1=0; proc2=0; proc3=0; proc4=0;
if proc=1 then proc1=1;
if proc=2 then proc2=1;
if proc=3 then proc3=1;
if proc=4 then proc4=1;

*****************
* Waiting times *
*****************;
 * number of weeks from registration on wait list to admission or removal ;
 weeks=intck('week',mdy(m,d,yo),
 mdy(month(adm_date),day(adm_date),year(adm_date)));
 * number of weeks from first date to registration on wait list ;
 week0=intck('week',mdy(6,1,1994),mdy(m,d,yo));

********************
* Wait-list status *
********************;
/* Status codes
   0 - Received surgery
   1 - Still on wait list
```

```
       2 - Cancellation of booked surgery due to patient condition
       3 - Patient condition prevented booking surgery
       4 - Health deterioration: stroke, rupture, tia
       5 - Death before admission
       6 - Patient refused to undergo booked surgery
       7 - Patient improved
       8 - Patient decided against surgery
  */
  status=0;if taken_of^=. then status=taken_of;
  * assign status "still on wait list" to patients with delays over 1 year *;
  * those who are active already have 'WL' in adm_wit and will not be affected *;
  if adm_wit='' then do;
    adm_wit='WL';
    weeks=53;
    status=1;
    if_not=6;
  end;
  wait=weeks;


  **********************************************
  * Admission within/beyond target access time *
  **********************************************;
  * correct adm_wit if wait<=gl among received ;
  if wait<=gl and adm_wit='No' then do;
    adm_wit='Yes';
    if_not=0;
  end;
  * correct adm_wit if wait>gl among received ;
  if wait>gl and adm_wit='Yes' then do;
    adm_wit='No';
    if_not=1;
  end;
 * correct wait if wait<=gl but there is info on if_not among removed ;
  if wait<=gl and adm_wit='N/A' and if_not>0 then do;
     wait=gl+1;
  end;
  if if_not=. then do;
    if adm_wit='Yes' then if_not=0;
    if adm_wit='No' then if_not=1;
    if adm_wit='N/A' then do;
      if wait <=gl then if_not=0;
      if wait >gl then if_not=1;
      if wait >gl and proc=4 then if_not=6;
    end;
 end;
run;
```

SAS Code B.2: DATA step to censor waiting times

```
/***********************************************************
 * Program: \vascular\sas\common\step_2.sas
 *
 * Input data: "vasc2"
 *
 * Description: DATA step to censor waiting times
 *
 ***********************************************************/

data vasc;
  set vasc2;
  status0=status;
  if wait>40 then do; /* censor if wait is more than 40 weeks */
    wait=41;
    if adm_wit='N/A' or weeks>40 then do;
      adm_wit='WL';
    end;
    status=1;
  end;

  **********
  * Outcome *
  **********;
  outcome=1; * surgery or censored within target access time ;
  if adm_wit='No' or adm_wit='WL' or adm_wit='N/A' then do;
    outcome=2;
      /* no surgery within target time due to patient problems */
    if if_not=3 or if_not=4 or if_not=5 then outcome=3;
      /* no surgery within target time due to hospital problems */
    if if_not=6 then outcome=4;
      /* no surgery within target time due to doctor decision */
    if if_not=7 then outcome=5;
      /* no surgery within target time due to the length of wait list */
  end;
  if adm_wit='N/A' then do;
    if wait<gl or if_not=0 then outcome=1; * censored within target time ;
  end;

  ******************
  * Delay indicator *
  ******************;
  del=0;
  if outcome=2|outcome=3|outcome=4 then del=1;
run;
```

B.1.2 Preparing data set on access to coronary artery bypass grafting surgery

SAS Code B.3: DATA step to create analytical data set

```
/**********************************************************
 * Program: \cabg\sas\common\step_1.sas
 *
 * Input data: "booklib" is a library that contains
 *  the data set "cabg1" of original records
 *
 * Description: DATA step to apply exclusion criteria,
 * create categorical and indicator variables,
 * and compute waiting times
 **********************************************************/

data cabg2;
  set booklib.cabg1;
  /* Exclusion criteria
     patients:
     - with emergency priority status at registration
     - who received surgery within one day and arrived on weekend
     - with reason for removal of surgery done, no OR report
     - who arrived and were removed from wait list on same date
  */
  where ur_bk^='0'
        & ^( (wl_rm='0'|wl_rm='10') & (weekday(wl_st)=7 | weekday(wl_st)=1)
          & intck('day',mdy(month(wl_st),day(wl_st),year(wl_st)),
          mdy(month(wl_en),day(wl_en),year(wl_en)))=1 )
        & wl_rm^='6'
        & wl_st^=wl_en;
  by bccr_id;


  *******************
  * Priority groups *
  *******************;
  * indicator for priority group at registration ;
  iurbk1=0; iurbk2=0; iurbk3=0; iurbku=0;
  if ur_bk='1' then do; iurbk1=1; end;
  if ur_bk='2' then do; iurbk2=1; end;
  if ur_bk='3' then do; iurbk3=1; end;
  if ur_bk='U' then do; iurbku=1; end;


  *************
  * Age groups *
  *************;
  * collapse age categories ;
  agecat2=99; age0=0; age1=0; age2=0; age3=0; age4=0;
  if age<50 then do; agecat2=0; age0=1; end;
  if age>=50 & age<60 then do; agecat2=1; age1=1; end;
  if age>=60 & age<70 then do; agecat2=2; age2=1; end;
  if age>=70 & age<80 then do; agecat2=3; age3=1; end;
```

```
if age>=80 then do; agecat2=4; age4=1; end;
if age=. then do; agecat2=99; end;


***********************
* Registration period *
***********************;
* registration period and indicator variables ;
cy=99;
icy91=0; icy93=0; icy95=0; icy97=0; icy99=0; icy01=0;
if wl_yr='1991' | wl_yr='1992' then do; cy=1; icy91=1; end;
if wl_yr='1993' | wl_yr='1994' then do; cy=2; icy93=1; end;
if wl_yr='1995' | wl_yr='1996' then do; cy=3; icy95=1; end;
if wl_yr='1997' | wl_yr='1998' then do; cy=4; icy97=1; end;
if wl_yr='1999' | wl_yr='2000' then do; cy=5; icy99=1; end;
* split into first 3 years vs last 2 years ;
icy=99;
if cy=1 | cy=2 | cy=3 then icy=0;
if cy=4 | cy=5 then icy=1;


*******
* Sex *
*******;
sexfn=0;  * numeric indicator for sex ;
if sexf='0' then sexfn=0;
if sexf='1' then sexfn=1;
if sexf='U' then sexfn=.;


***************
* Comorbidity *
***************;
* comorbidity categorical variable ;
comor=99; icmc1=0; icmc2=0; icmc3=0;
if cm_ch='0' then do; comor=1; icmc1=1; end; * none ;
if cm_ch^='0' & cm_bk='0' then do; comor=2; icmc2=1; end; * no major == minor;
if cm_ch^='0' & cm_bk='1' then do; comor=3; icmc3=1; end; * major ;


************
* Hospital *
************;
* numeric indicators for institution at registration ;
ihsp1=0; ihsp2=0; ihsp3=0; ihsp4=0;
if inst_bk='1' then ihsp1=1;
if inst_bk='2' then ihsp2=1;
if inst_bk='3' then ihsp3=1;
if inst_bk='4' then ihsp4=1;


*******************
* Coronary anatomy *
*******************;
* collapse anatomy categories ;
```

```
anatom2='99';
if anatom='1' then anatom2='1'; * left main ;
if anatom='2' | anatom='3' | anatom='5' then anatom2='2'; * multivessel ;
if anatom='4' | anatom='U' then anatom2='3'; * limited ;


*****************
* Waiting times *
*****************;
* number of calendar weeks from January 1, 1991 to registration on wait list ;
week0=intck('week',mdy(1,1,1991),mdy(month(wl_st),day(wl_st),year(wl_st)));
* weeks on wait list ;
wait=intck('week',mdy(month(wl_st),day(wl_st),year(wl_st)),
    mdy(month(wl_en),day(wl_en),year(wl_en)));
* months on wait list ;
waitm=intck('month',mdy(month(wl_st),day(wl_st),year(wl_st)),
    mdy(month(wl_en),day(wl_en),year(wl_en)));
* target access times ;
mrwt=999;
if ur_bk='1' then mrwt=0.5; * urgent, target time < 1 week;
if ur_bk='2' then mrwt=6; * semiurgent, target time <= 6 weeks;
if ur_bk='3' then mrwt=12; * nonurgent, target time <= 12 weeks;
* indicator for removal within target access time ;
iadw=0;
if wait<=mrwt then iadw=1; * removal within target time ;
if mrwt=999 then iadw=99; * emergency or missing cases ;


********************
* Wait-list status *
********************;
status=99; * status indicator in numeric format ;
if wl_rm='0' then status=0; * underwent surgery ;
if wl_rm='1' then status=1; * died ;
if wl_rm='2' then status=2; * medical treatment ;
if wl_rm='3' then status=3; * patient request ;
if wl_rm='4' then status=4; * transferred ;
if wl_rm='5' then status=5; * otherwise removed from list ;
if wl_rm='6' then status=6; * surgery done, no OR report ;
if wl_rm='7' then status=7; * wait list ;
if wl_rm='8' then status=8; * other surgery (for valve replacement, etc) ;
if wl_rm='9' then status=1; * patient died (no corresponding vital statistics);
if wl_rm='10' then status=12; * unplanned emergency admission ;
if (wl_rm='0' | wl_rm='10') & wait=0 then status=13; * immediate sx ;


**************
* Death dates *
**************;
* preserve original death date ;
dthdate0=dthdate;
* refine death dates ;
* refine death dates among those who died in hospital ;
```

```
if exit_code='X' then dthdate=sepdate;
* refine death dates among those who died on WL ;
if wl_rm='1' | wl_rm='9' then dthdate=wl_en;
* if discharged alive but sepdate before dthdate then refine dthdate ;
if (wl_rm='0'|wl_rm='10') & exit_code^='X' & dthdate^=. & (sepdate>dthdate) then
  dthdate=intnx('day',sepdate,1);

*****************************
* Perioperative death times *
*****************************;
* months from registration on wait list to death or end of study ;
twlsdthm=.;
if dthdate^=. then do;
  twlsdthm=intck('month',mdy(month(wl_st),day(wl_st),year(wl_st)),
  mdy(month(dthdate),day(dthdate),year(dthdate)));
end;
if dthdate=. then do;
  twlsdthm=intck('month',mdy(month(wl_st),day(wl_st),year(wl_st)),
  mdy(12,31,2002));
end;

****************
* Death status *
****************;
dthsts=99;
* preoperative death on wait list ;
if (wl_rm='1'|wl_rm='9') & wait<=52 then dthsts=1;
* in-hospital death ;
if (wl_rm='0' | wl_rm='10') & dthdate^=. & exit_code='X' then dthsts=2;
* late postoperative death ;
if (wl_rm='0' | wl_rm='10') & dthdate^=. & exit_code^='X' then dthsts=3;
* death after removal from wait list without surgery ;
if ^(wl_rm='0'|wl_rm='10') & ^((wl_rm='1'|wl_rm='9') & wait<=52)
  & dthdate^=. then dthsts=4;
* alive at study end ;
if dthdate=. & ^(wl_rm='9') then dthsts=98;
run;
```

SAS Code B.4: DATA step to censor waiting times

```
/*****************************************************
 * Program: \cabg\sas\common\step_2.sas
 *
 * Input data: "cabg2"
 *
 * Description: DATA step to censor waiting times
 *****************************************************/
```

```
data cabg;
  set cabg2;
  ptno=_N_;
  ************************
  * Censor waiting times *
  ************************;
  wait0=wait;
  waitm0=waitm;
  status0=status;
  status5y=status;

  * censor if wait is more than 52 weeks ;
  if wait>52 then do;
    wait=53;
    status=9;
  end;

  wait05=wait;
  if wait=0 then wait05=0.5;

  * censor if wait is more than 60 months ;
  if waitm>60 then do;
    waitm=61;
    status5y=9;
  end;

  *************
  * Indicator *
  *************;
  * indicator for wait-list death ;
  death=0; if status=1 then death=1;

  **********************
  * Censor death times *
  **********************;
  twlsdthcm=twlsdthm;
  dthstssc=dthsts;

  * censor if transferred or underwent other surgery ;
  if status0=4|status0=8 then do;
    twlsdthcm=waitm0;
    dthstssc=99; * alive, censored ;
  end;

  * censor if time is more than 5 years;
  if twlsdthcm>60 then do;
    twlsdthcm=61;
    dthstssc=99; * alive, censored ;
  end;
run;
```

B.1.3 Preparing data set on access to cholecystectomy surgery

SAS Code B.5: DATA step to create analytical data set

```
/*********************************************************
 * Program: \chole\sas\common\step_1.sas
 *
 * Input data: "booklib" is a library that contains
 *  the data set "chole1" of original records
 *
 * Description: DATA step to create categorical
 *  and indicator variables
 *********************************************************/

data chole2;
  set booklib.chole1;

  ******************
  * Age categories *
  *****************;
  /* indicator variables for age group */
  ag1=(ag_ca1=1);
  ag2=(ag_ca1=2);
  ag3=(ag_ca1=3);
  ag4=(ag_ca1=4);
  ag5=(ag_ca1=5);
  ag6=(ag_ca1=6);
  ag7=(ag_ca1=7);

  *******
  * Sex *
  *******;
  sexm=1-sexf;

  **********************
  * Registration period *
  *********************;
  * indicator variables for registration period ;
  fy1=(ep1=1); fy2=(ep1=2); fy3=(ep1=3);

  ****************************
  * Surgeon annual case volume *
  ***************************;
  * indicator variables for surgeon volume ;
  vt1=(vt=1); vt2=(vt=2); vt3=(vt=3);
run;
```

```
/**********************************************************
 * Program: \chole\sas\common\step_2.sas
 *
 * Input data: "chole2"
 *
 * Description: DATA step to create patient-interval data
 **********************************************************/
data chole;
  array p[7] per1-per7;
  array lp[7] lpr1-lpr7;
  set chole2;
  **************************
  * Waiting-time intervals *
  **************************;
  /* number of weeks in interval */
  per1=3; per2=4; per3=4; per4=8; per5=8; per6=12; per7=12;
  /* lowerbound of interval */
  lpr1=0; lpr2=3; lpr3=7; lpr4=11; lpr5=19; lpr6=27; lpr7=39;

  **********************
  * Waiting-time period *
  **********************;
  per=(wait>0)+(wait>=4)+(wait>=8)+(wait>=12)+
      (wait>=20)+(wait>=28)+(wait>=40);

  *********************************
  * Time-dependent event indicator *
  *********************************;
  do j=1 to per;
    emgadm=0; * indicator for emergency admission ;
    eladm=0; * indicator for elective admission ;
    tim=p[j];
    if j=per then do;
      tim=wait-lp[j];
      emgadm=(event=2);
      eladm=(event=1);
    end;
     * offset variable for Poisson regression ;
     ltim=log(tim);
     * indicator variables for waiting-time interval ;
     wcat1=(j=1); wcat2=(j=2); wcat3=(j=3); wcat4=(j=4); wcat5=(j=5);
     wcat6=(j=6); wcat7=(j=7);
     output;
  end;
run;
```

B.2 Estimating summary measures

B.2.1 Macro to estimate proportion by group

SAS Code B.6: Macro to estimate event proportions by group

```
/*********************************************************
 * Program: macro_getprop.sas
 *
 * Description: 'getprop' is a macro to compute event proportions by group
 *
 *  Input:
 *    dat, specifies the name of the data set
 *    grp, group variable in 'dat'
 *    sts, status variable in 'dat' for status of patient
 *    rcdc, corresponding 'sts' code for patients who
 *        experienced event of interest
 *    alp, number between 0 and 1; 100(1-alp)% confidence interval
 *        estimated for event proportion
 *    outdat, name of output data set
 *
 *  Output:
 *    data set called 'outdat' with columns for the following:
 *      grp, grouping variable
 *      numpt, number of patients
 *      totev, total number of events
 *      evprop, event proportion (=totev/numpt*100)
 *      seevprop, standard error of estimated event proportion
 *          (approx sqrt(evprop/100*(1-evprop/100)/numpt)*100 )
 *      lbprop, lowerbound of 100*(1-alp)% CI for event proportion
 *      ubprop, upperbound of 100*(1-alp)% CI for event proportion
 *
 * Developed by Lisa Kuramoto (2003/12/09);
 * Revised by Lisa Kuramoto (2004/04/27);
 * Revised by Lisa Kuramoto (2004/05/03);
 * Revised by Lisa Kuramoto (2006/09/22);
 * Revised by Lisa Kuramoto (2006/09/25);
 *********************************************************/

%macro getprop(dat,grp,sts,rcdc,alp,outdat);
  * create indicator for event of interest *;
  data evind;
    set &dat;
    ev=0;
    if &sts=&rcdc then ev=1;
  run;

  * compute total number of events by group *;
  proc sort data=evind out=evinds;
    by &grp;
  run;
```

```
proc means noprint nway data=evinds;
  by &grp;
  var ev;
  output out=evot
         sum=totev;
run;

* compute event proportion *;
data &outdat;
  set evot;
  * event proportion and standard error *;
  evprop=totev/_FREQ_;
  seevprop=sqrt(evprop*(1-evprop)/_FREQ_);

  * approximate 100(1-alp)% CI for event proportion *;
  lbprop=evprop-probit(1-&alp/2)*seevprop;
  ubprop=evprop+probit(1-&alp/2)*seevprop;

  * report as percentage *;
  evprop=evprop*100; seevprop=seevprop*100;
  lbprop=lbprop*100;
  ubprop=ubprop*100;

  rename _FREQ_=numpt;
  drop _TYPE_;
run;

proc print data=&outdat;
  format evprop 8.1 seevprop 8.1 lbprop 8.1 ubprop 8.1;
run;
%mend getprop;
```

B.2.2 Macro to estimate event rates by group

SAS Code B.7: Macro to estimate event rates by group

```
/********************************************************
 * Program: macro_getrate.sas
 *
 * Description: "getrate" is a macro to compute event rates by group
 *
 * Input:
 *   dat - specifies the name of the data set
 *   grp - group variable in dat
 *   time - waiting time variable in dat
 *   sts - status variable in dat for status of patient
 *   rcdc - corresponding sts code for patients who
 *       experienced event of interest
 *   unit - integer number to estimate
```

```
*    event rate per unit patient-times
*    alp - number between 0 and 1 to estimate
*    100(1-alp)% confidence interval for event rate
*    outdat - name of output data set
*
* Output:
*    data set "outdat" with columns
*      grp - grouping variable
*      numpt - number of patients
*      totev - total number of events
*      totpttme - total number of patient-times
*      evrt - event rate (=totev/totpttme)
*      seaevrt - standard error of estimated event rate
*         (approx sqrt(totev)/totpttme )
*      lbrt - lowerbound of 100*(1-alp)% CI for event rate
*      ubrt - upperbound of 100*(1-alp)% CI for event rate
*
* Developed by Lisa Kuramoto (2003/12/09)
* Revised by Lisa Kuramoto (2004/04/27)
* Revised by Lisa Kuramoto (2004/05/03)
* Revised by Lisa Kuramoto (2006/09/20)
******************************************************/

%macro getrate(dat,grp,time,sts,rcdc,unit,alp,outdat);
  /* create indicator for event of interest */
  data evind;
    set &dat;
    ev=0;
    if &sts=&rcdc then ev=1;
  run;
  /* compute total number of events and patient-time by group */
  proc sort data=evind out=evinds;
    by &grp;
  run;
  proc means noprint nway data=evinds;
    by &grp;
    var ev &time;
    output out=evrate
           sum=totev totpttme;
  run;
  /* compute event rate */
  data &outdat;
    set evrate;
    /* event rate and standard error */
    evrt=totev/totpttme*&unit;
    seevrt=sqrt(totev)/totpttme*&unit;
    /* approximate 100(1-alp)% CI for event rate */
    lbrt=evrt-probit(1-&alp/2)*seevrt;
    ubrt=evrt+probit(1-&alp/2)*seevrt;
    rename _FREQ_=numpt;
```

```
   drop _TYPE_;
 run;
 proc print data=&outdat;
   format evrt 8.2 seevrt 8.2 lbrt 8.2 ubrt 8.2;
 run;
%mend getrate;
```

B.3 Creating new variables and reformatting records

B.3.1 DATA step for estimating wait-list size

SAS Code B.8: DATA step to estimate wait-list size

```
/*******************************************************
 * Program: \cabg\sas\common\wlsize.sas
 *
 * Input data:  "cabg2"
 *
 * Description: DATA step to compute wait-list size
 *******************************************************/

* find number of surgeries by calendar week and hospital *;
data cabg2u;
  set cabg2;

  * classify patients with unknown priority at booking *;
  ur_bk2=ur_bk;
  if ur_bk='U' & (ur_sx='1' | ur_sx='2' | ur_sx='3') then ur_bk2=ur_sx;
  if ur_bk='U' & (ur_sx='U' | ur_sx='N/A') then ur_bk2='3';
  if ur_bk='U' & ur_sx='0' then ur_bk2='3';

run;

* patients who were on surgical wait list during study period *;
data sub;
  set cabg2u;

  * calendar week of registration on wait list from fixed date *;
  week1=intck('week',mdy(1,1,1990),mdy(month(wl_st),day(wl_st),year(wl_st)));

  * calendar week of removal from wait list from fixed date *;
  week2=intck('week',mdy(1,1,1990),mdy(month(wl_en),day(wl_en),year(wl_en)));

run;

* expand to patient-week data *;
* only include weeks that contribute to wait-list size *;
data subex;
  set sub;

  * do not contribute to wait-list size during week of arrival *;
  week1p1=week1+1;

  * do not contribute to wait-list size during week of removal/surgery *;
  week2m1=(wl_rm^='7')*(week2-1)+(wl_rm='7')*week2;

  * contribute to wait-list size from week after registration *;
  * to just before removal from WL *;
```

```
  do i=week1p1 to week2m1;
    cweek=i;
    output;
  end;

run;


* count number of surgeries by hospital, calendar week *;
* and priority at registration *;
ods output Table=sztbl;
proc tabulate data=subex missing ;
  class inst_bk cweek ur_bk2;
  table inst_bk*cweek*ur_bk2;
run;


* compute wait-list size by priority within each hospital *;
* assumes higher priority undergo surgery first *;
data sztbl2;
  set sztbl;
  by inst_bk cweek;
  retain wlsize;

  if first.cweek then wlsize=0;

  if N=. then N=0;

  wlsize=wlsize+N;

  rename cweek=week1; * week of registration on surgical WL *;
  keep inst_bk cweek ur_bk2 wlsize;
run;


* extract patients with referral date during study period of interest *;
* and who are on surgical WL *;
proc sort data=sub out=subs;
  by inst_bk week1 ur_bk2;
run;


* merge data with WL size data *;
data wlszdat;
  * append new variable 'wlsize' to data set *;
  merge subs (in=ori) sztbl2;
  by inst_bk week1 ur_bk2;

  * those at beginning of study period defined to have 0 wlsize *;
  if wlsize=. then wlsize=0;

  * create 4 categories of wait-list size *;
  * (dependent upon hospital at booking) *;
  wlszcat=0;
```

```
wlsz1=0; wlsz2=0; wlsz3=0; wlsz4=0;
if (inst_bk='1' | inst_bk='2' | inst_bk='4') &
  wlsize>=0 & wlsize<=14 then do; wlszcat=1; wlsz1=1; end;
if (inst_bk='1' | inst_bk='2' | inst_bk='4') &
  wlsize>=15 & wlsize<=29 then do; wlszcat=2; wlsz2=1; end;
if (inst_bk='1' | inst_bk='2' | inst_bk='4') &
  wlsize>=30 & wlsize<=59 then do; wlszcat=3; wlsz3=1; end;
if (inst_bk='1' | inst_bk='2' | inst_bk='4') &
  wlsize>=60 then do; wlszcat=4; wlsz4=1; end;

if inst_bk='3' & wlsize>=0 & wlsize<=24 then do; wlszcat=1; wlsz1=1; end;
if inst_bk='3' & wlsize>=25 & wlsize<=49 then do; wlszcat=2; wlsz2=1; end;
if inst_bk='3' & wlsize>=50 & wlsize<=99 then do; wlszcat=3; wlsz3=1; end;
if inst_bk='3' & wlsize>=100 then do; wlszcat=4; wlsz4=1; end;

if ori=1 then output;
run;
proc sort data=wlszdat;
  by bccr_id;
run;

* censor waiting times after 52 weeks *;
data wtimesz2;
  set wlszdat;

  ptno=_N_;

  * retain original status *;
  status0=status;

  * censor if wait is more than 52;
  if wait>52 then do;
    wait=53;
    status=9;
  end;

  wait05=wait;
  if wait=0 then wait05=0.5;

run;
```

B.3.2 DATA step for creating patient by week data for access to surgery

SAS Code B.9: DATA step to create patient by week data for access to surgery

```
/*******************************************************
 * Program: \cabg\sas\common\ptwkdata_access.sas
 *
 * Input data: "wtimesz2"
```

```
*
* Description: DATA step to create patient by week data for access to surgery
*******************************************************/

data wtimeszex;
  set wtimesz2;
  retain cweek;

  do time=0 to wait;

     access=0; * access to surgery indicator *;
     if time=wait and (status=0|status=13) then access=1;

     * create calendar week variable *;
     if time=0 then cweek=week0+1;
     if time^=0 then cweek=cweek+1;

     if time=0 then time=0.5;
     if time<=52 then output;
     if time=0.5 then time=0;
  end;

run;
```

B.3.3 DATA step for creating patient by week data for on-time surgery

SAS Code B.10: DATA step to create patient by week data for on-time surgery

```
/********************************************************
* Program: \cabg\sas\common\ptwkdata_ontime.sas
*
* Input data: "wtimesz2"
*
* Description: DATA step to create patient by week data for on-time surgery
*******************************************************/

data wtimeszex2;
  set wtimesz2;
  retain cweek;

  do time=0 to wait;

     access=0; * access to surgery indicator *;
     if time=wait and (status=0|status=13) then access=1;

     * create calendar week variable *;
     if time=0 then cweek=week0+1;
     if time^=0 then cweek=cweek+1;
```

```
    if time=0 then time=0.5;
      if (ur_bk2='1' & time<=0.5) | (ur_bk2='2' & time<=6) |
      (ur_bk2='3' & time<=12) then output;
    if time=0.5 then time=0;
  end;

run;
```

B.3.4 DATA step for expansion to pseudovalues data

SAS Code B.11: DATA step to create pseudovalue data

```
/********************************************************
 * Program: \cabg\sas\common\pvdata.sas
 *
 * Input data: "cabg"
 *
 * Description: DATA step to create pseudovalue data (no censored observations)
 ********************************************************/

data cabg23ex2;
  set cabg;
  where ur_bk='2'|ur_bk='3';
  by ptno;
  retain psvalue;

  if first.ptno then do;
    psvalue=0; * pseudovalue *;
  end;

  * pseudovalues for CIF of death *;
  do i=0 to 52;
    time=i;
    if time=0 then time=0.5;
    if status=1 & time>=wait05 then psvalue=1;
    output;
  end;

  keep wait05 ur_bk status ptno time psvalue
  iurbk1 iurbk2 iurbk3 iurbku
  sexfn
  age0 age1 age2 age3 age4
  icy91 icy93 icy95 icy97 icy99
  icmc1 icmc2 icmc3
  ihsp1 ihsp2 ihsp3 ihsp4
  ;
run;
```

C

Matlab code

C.1 Estimating the cumulative incidence function

Matlab Code C.1: Function to estimate cumulative incidence function for the event of interest

```
%% 'getcif' is a function to compute the cumulative incidence
%%         for event of interest
%%
%% Input:
%%    N, total number at risk (integer)
%%    e, number of events of interest at current time point
%%       (vector of integers)
%%    r, number of competing events at current time point
%%       (vector of integers)
%%    c, number of censored observations at current time point
%%       (vector of integers)
%%    t, distinct, ordered times (vector of integers/doubles)
%%
%%      Note that the elements of 'e', 'r', and 'c' should
%%      correspond to the same time points in 't'.
%%
%% Output:
%%   F, estimated cumulative incidence function for event of
%%      interest at each time point in 't'
%% varF, estimate variance of cumulative incidence function for
%%      event of interest at each time point in 't'
%% t, distinct, ordered times (vector of integers/doubles)
%% n, number at risk *beyond* time point
%%
%% Developed by Lisa Kuramoto (2004/08/18);
%% Reviewed by Boris Sobolev (2004/09/01);
%% Revised by Lisa Kuramoto (2005/05/20).
%%
%% Based on Kalbfleisch and Prentice (1980) and Gaynor (1993).

function [F, varF, t, n] = getcif(N,e,r,c,t)
```

```matlab
%% estimate cumulative incidence function %%

% number of distinct, ordered time points
ntme=length(e);

% number at risk beyond time point
n=N-cumsum(sum([e r c],2));

% number at risk at time point
Y=[N; n(1:(ntme-1))];

% total number of events at time point
dd=e+r;

% hazard of event of interest
lam=e./Y;

% overall survival
pS=1-dd./Y;
pS=[1; pS];
pS=pS(1:(length(pS)-1));
S=cumprod(pS);

% cumulative incidence for event of interest
F=cumsum(lam.*S);


%% estimate variance of cumulative incidence function %%

% estimated survival function
tmp2=[1; cumprod(1+(c(1:(ntme-1)))./n(1:(ntme-1)))];
KMc=cumsum(dd.*tmp2)/N;
if any(isnan(KMc))
   indx=ntme-sum(isnan(KMc));
   KMc(isnan(KMc))=KMc(indx);
end;
S=1-KMc;
S=[1; S];
S=S(1:(length(S)-1));

% covariance matrix of lamS
ny=length(Y)-1;
tmp=dd(1:ny)./(Y(1:ny).*(Y(1:ny)-dd(1:ny)));
sumtmp=cumsum(tmp);
sumtmp=[0; sumtmp];

lamS=lam.*S;

vlamS=zeros(ntme,1);
```

```
ind=(e~=0);
vlamS(ind)=lamS(ind).^2.*((Y(ind)-e(ind))./(e(ind).*Y(ind))+sumtmp(ind));

covmtx=zeros(ntme,ntme);
tmpmtx=zeros(ntme,ntme);
for i=1:(ntme-1),
   for j=(i+1):ntme,
       ind=(e(i)~=0 & e(j)~=0);
       covmtx(i,j)=ind*lamS(i)*lamS(j)*(-1/Y(i)+sumtmp(i));
       covmtx(j,i)=covmtx(i,j);
       tmpmtx(i,j)=covmtx(i,j);
   end;
   covmtx(i,i)=vlamS(i);
end;
covmtx(ntme,ntme)=vlamS(ntme);


% compute variance of F
crstrm=sum(tmpmtx,1)';
varF=cumsum(vlamS)+2*cumsum(crstrm);
```

C.2 Estimating the conditional probability function

Matlab Code C.2: Function to estimate conditional probability function for the event of interest

```
%% 'getcp' is a function to compute the conditional probability
%%          function for event of interest
%%
%% Input:
%%    N, total number at risk (integer)
%%    e, number of events of interest at current time point
%%       (vector of integers)
%%    r, number of competing events at current time point
%%       (vector of integers)
%%    c, number of censored observations at current time point
%%       (vector of integers)
%%    t, distinct, ordered times (vector of integers/doubles)
%%
%%      Note that the elements of 'e', 'r', and 'c' should
%%      correspond to the same time points in 't'.
%%
%% Output:
%%      CP, estimated conditional probability function for event
%%          of interest at each time point in 't' (vector of doubles)
%%      varCP, estimated variance of conditional probability
%%          function for event of interest at each time point
%%          in 't' (vector of doubles)
%%      t, distinct, ordered times (vector of integers/doubles)
```

```
%%
%% Helper function:
%%      'getcif' to compute the cumulative incidence function
%%
%% Developed by Lisa Kuramoto (2004/08/13);
%% Reviewed by Boris Sobolev (2004/08/27);
%% Revised by Lisa Kuramoto (2004/08/18);
%% Revised Lisa Kuramoto (2006/12/07).
%%
%% Based on Pepe (1993).

function [CP, varCP, t] = getcp(N,e,r,c,t)

%% estimate conditional probability function %%

% number of distinct, ordered time points
ntme=length(e);

% cumulative incidence for event of interest
[F1 varF1 t1 n1] = getcif(N,e,r,c,t);

% cumulative incidence for competing event
[F2 varF2 t2 n2] = getcif(N,r,e,c,t);

% conditional probabilities for event of interest
CP=F1./(1-F2);

% find number at risk beyond time point *
n=N-cumsum(sum([e r c],2));

%% estimate variance for conditional probability function %%

% number at risk at time point
Y=[N; n(1:(ntme-1))];

% overall survival
[Fo varFo to no] = getcif(N,e+r,zeros(length(e),1),c,t);
S=1-Fo;

% variance of CP
trm1=S.^2./(1-F2).^4;
num=(1-F2).^2.*e + F1.^2.*r;
den=Y.*(Y-1);
smd=num./den;
cs=cumsum(smd);

varCP=trm1.*cs;
```

C.3 Comparing conditional probability functions in two groups

Matlab Code C.3: Function to compare conditional probability functions in two groups

```
%% "cptest" is a function to compare the conditional probability
%%          functions between group 1 and 2
%%
%% Input:
%%    dat1, nt by 4 matrix for group 1, where 'nt' is the number
%%          of unique time points and columns are as follows:
%%               (1) waiting time
%%               (2) number of events of interest
%%               (3) number of censored observations
%%               (4) number of competing events
%%    dat2, nt by 4 matrix for group 2, where 'nt' is the number
%%          of unique time points and columns are as follows:
%%               (1) waiting time
%%               (2) number of events of interest
%%               (3) number of censored observations
%%               (4) number of competing events
%%    rho, exponent for the weight function
%%      rho=0 => weight of 1 for all time points;
%%      rho=1 => weight equal to censored distribution
%%
%% Output:
%%    del, "difference" between CP in group 1 and 2
%%    sig2, estimated variance of "difference"
%%    tstat, test statistic (=del/sqrt(sig2))
%%    pval, p-value
%%    W, weight function
%%
%% Helper functions:
%%    - getcif.m
%%
%% Restrictions:
%%    - assumes the difference between time points is 1 %
%%    - assumes observed time points for group 1 are same as group 2
%%    - compares across first 53 time points
%%
%% Developed by Lisa Kuramoto (2004/08/13);
%% Reviewed by Boris Sobolev (2004/08);
%% Revised by Lisa Kuramoto (2006/12/07);
%%
%% Based on Pepe (1993).

function [del, sig2, tstat, pval, W] = cptest(dat1,dat2,rho)

% group 1 ;
wt1=dat1(:,1); % waiting time
e1=dat1(:,2); % number of events of interest
c1=dat1(:,3); % number of censored
```

```
r1=dat1(:,4); % number of competing events
N1=sum(e1)+sum(r1)+sum(c1); % number initially at risk

% group 2 ;
wt2=dat2(:,1); % waiting time
e2=dat2(:,2); % number of events of interest
c2=dat2(:,3); % number of censored
r2=dat2(:,4); % number of competing events
N2=sum(e2)+sum(r2)+sum(c2); % number initially at risk

N=N1+N2; % total number initially at risk;

zros=zeros(length(wt1),1);

%% non-parametric estimates of cumulative incidence function %%
% cumulative incidence for event of interest in group 1
[F1I v t1I n1] = getcif(N1,e1,r1,c1,wt1); F1I=F1I(1:53);
% cumulative incidence for competing event in group 1
[F2I v t2I n1] = getcif(N1,r1,e1,c1,wt1); F2I=F2I(1:53);

% cumulative incidence for event of interest in group 2
[F1II v t1II n2] = getcif(N2,e2,r2,c2,wt2); F1II=F1II(1:53);
% cumulative incidence for competing event in group 2
[F2II v t2II n2] = getcif(N2,r2,e2,c2,wt2); F2II=F2II(1:53);

%% non-parametric estimates of conditional probability function %%
% conditional probability of event of interest
CP1I=F1I./(1-F2I);    % CP for event of interest in group 1
CP1II=F1II./(1-F2II); % CP for event of interest in group 2

%% non-parametric estimates of complement Kaplan-Meier function %%
% group 1
cns=e1+r1;
[CKMcI v tmp2 n1] = getcif(N1,c1,zros,cns,wt1); CKMcI=CKMcI(1:53);
CKMI=1-CKMcI;
% group 2
cns=e2+r2;
[CKMcII v tmp2 n2] = getcif(N2,c2,zros,cns,wt2); CKMcII=CKMcII(1:53);
CKMII=1-CKMcII;

%% non-parametric estimates of S (ie. overall survival) %%
[ScI tmp tmp2 tmp3] = getcif(N1,e1+r1,zros,c1,wt1);
SI=1-ScI(1:53);
[ScII tmp tmp2 tmp3] = getcif(N2,e2+r2,zros,c2,wt2);
SII=1-ScII(1:53);

%% number at risk just before time t %%
y1=[N1; n1];
y2=[N2; n2];
```

```
%%% Compute test statistic to compare the CIFs from two samples %%%
%%% H0: CP_1==CP_2
%%% HA: CP_1>=CP_2 if W>0

%% Compute weights %%
num=CKMI.*CKMII;
den=(N1/N)*CKMI + (N2/N)*CKMII;
W=(num./den).^rho;

tmp=[0; wt1(1:53)]; % assuming wt1=wt2;
tmediff=diff(tmp);

del=sqrt(N1*N2/N)*sum(W.*(CP1I-CP1II).*tmediff);


%% Compute variance %%
% group 1 %
Nt=length(wt1)-1; % number of time points
sig2I=0;          %variance

num=(1-F2I).^2.*e1(1:Nt) + F1I.^2.*r1(1:Nt);
den=y1(1:Nt).*(y1(1:Nt)-1);
trm2=num./den;
smd=W.*SI./(1-F2I).^2;

for k=1:Nt,
   trm1=sum(smd(k:Nt).*tmediff(k:Nt));
   sig2I = sig2I + trm1^2*trm2(k);
end;
sig2I=sig2I*N1;

% group 2 %
Nt=length(wt2)-1; % number of time points
sig2II=0;          %variance

num=(1-F2II).^2.*e2(1:Nt) + F1II.^2.*r2(1:Nt);
den=y2(1:Nt).*(y2(1:Nt)-1);
trm2=num./den;
smd=W.*SII./(1-F2II).^2;

for k=1:Nt,
   trm1=sum(smd(k:Nt).*tmediff(k:Nt));
   sig2II = sig2II + trm1^2*trm2(k);
end;
sig2II=sig2II*N2;


%% Compute estimated variance %%
sig2=(N2/N)*sig2I + (N1/N)*sig2II;
```

```
%% Compute test statistic %%
tstat=del/sqrt(sig2);

%% Compute p-value %%
pval=1-normcdf(tstat);
```

References

[1] C. Alberti, F. Metivier, P. Landais, E. Thervet, C. Legendre, and S. Chevret. Improving estimates of event incidence over time in populations exposed to other events - application to three large databases. *Journal of Clinical Epidemiology*, 56:536–545, 2003.

[2] P. D. Allison. Discrete-time methods for the analysis of event histories. *Sociological Methodology*, pages 61–98, 1982.

[3] P. D. Allison. *Survival Analysis using SAS: A Practical Guide*. SAS Institute, 1st edition, 1995.

[4] P. D. Allison. *Logistic Regression using the SAS System: Theory and Application*. SAS Institute, 1st edition, 1999.

[5] D. A. Alter, A. S. Basinski, and C. D. Naylor. A survey of provider experiences and perceptions of preferential access to cardiovascular care in Ontario, Canada. *Annals of Internal Medicine*, 129: 567–572, 1998.

[6] D. A. Alter, A. S. Basinski, E. A. Cohen, and C. D. Naylor. Fairness in the coronary angiography queue. *Canadian Medical Association Journal*, 161:813–817, 1999.

[7] D. G. Altman and J. M. Bland. Time to event (survival) data. *British Medical Journal*, 317:468–469, 1998.

[8] P. K. Andersen, L. S. Hansen, and N. Keiding. Non- and semi-parametric estimation of transition probabilities from censored observation of a non-homogeneous markov process. *Scandinavian Journal of Statistics*, 18:153–167, 1991.

[9] P. K. Andersen, J. P. Klein, and S. Rosthoj. Generalised linear models for correlated pseudo-observations, with applications to multi-state models. *Biometrika*, 90:15–27, 2003.

[10] P. W. Armstrong. Unrepresentative, invalid and misleading: are waiting times for elective admission wrongly calculated? *Journal of Epidemiology and Biostatistics*, 5:117–123, 2000.

[11] P. W. Armstrong. First steps in analysing NHS waiting times: avoiding the 'stationary and closed population' fallacy. *Statistics in Medicine*, 19:2037–2051, 2000.

[12] G. R. Baker, P. G. Norton, V. Flintoft, R. Blais, A. Brown, J. Cox, E. Etchells, W. A. Ghali, P. Hebert, S. R. Majumdar, M. O'Beirne, L. Palacios-Derflingher, R. J. Reid, S. Sheps, and R. Tamblyn. The Canadian adverse events study: the incidence of adverse events among hospital patients in Canada. *Canadian Medical Association Journal*, 170:1678–1686, 2004.

[13] J. Benichou and M. H. Gail. Estimates of absolute cause-specific risk in cohort studies. *Biometrics*, 46:813–826, 1990.

[14] D. Bennett and J. Bion. ABC of intensive care: organisation of intensive care. *British Medical Journal*, 318:1468–1470, 1999.

[15] S. J. Bernstein, H. Rigter, B. Brorsson, L. H. Hilborne, L. L. Leape, A. P. Meijler, J. K. Scholma, and A. S. Nord. Waiting for coronary revascularization: a comparison between New York State, the Netherlands and Sweden. *Health Policy*, 42:15–27, 1997.

[16] J. T. Blake and M. W. Carter. Surgical process scheduling: a structured review. *Journal of the Society for Health Systems*, 5:17–30, 1997.

[17] J. M. Bland and D. G. Altman. Survival probabilities (the Kaplan-Meier method). *British Medical Journal*, 317:1572–1580, 1998.

[18] J. M. Bland and D. G. Altman. The logrank test. *British Medical Journal*, 328:1073, 2004.

[19] I. M. Bongers, J. B. van der Meer, J. van den Bos, and J. P. Mackenbach. Socio-economic differences in general practitioner and outpatient specialist care in the Netherlands: a matter of health insurance? *Social Science & Medicine*, 44:1161–1168, 1997.

[20] B. Bridgewater. Mortality data in adult cardiac surgery for named surgeons: retrospective examination of prospectively collected data on coronary artery surgery and aortic valve replacement. *British Medical Journal*, 330:506–510, 2005.

[21] J. Bryant and J. J. Dignam. Semiparametric models for cumulative incidence functions. *Biometrics*, 60:182–190, 2004.

[22] K. Bull and D. J. Spiegelhalter. Survival analysis in observational studies. *Statistics in Medicine*, 16: 1041–1074, 1997.

[23] Statistics Canada. *Canadian classification of diagnostic, therapeutic and surgical procedures*. Statistics Canada Health Division, 2nd edition, 1991.

[24] R. J. Caplan, T. F. Pajak, and J. D. Cox. Analysis of the probability and risk of cause-specific failure. *International Journal of Radiation Oncology Biology Physics*, 29:1183–1186, 1994.

[25] R. Chamberlayne, B. Green, M. L. Barer, C. Hertzman, W. J. Lawrence, and S. B. Sheps. Creating a population-based linked health database: a new resource for health services research. *Canadian Journal of Public Health*, 89:270–273, 1998.

[26] J. T. Christenson, F. Simonet, and M. Schmuziger. The influence of age on the outcome of primary coronary artery bypass grafting. *Journal of Cardiovascular Surgery (Torino)*, 40:333–338, 1999.

[27] K. A. Clover, T. A. Dobbins, T. J. Smyth, and R. W. Sanson-Fisher. Factors associated with waiting time for surgery. *The Medical Journal of Australia*, 169:464–468, 1998.

[28] L. H. Cohn and L. H. Jr Edmunds. *Cardiac Surgery in the Adult*. McGraw-Hill, 2003.

[29] T. Colton. *Statistics in Medicine*. Little, Brown and Company, 1st edition, 1974.

[30] A. Coulter, V. Seagroatt, and K. McPherson. Relation between general practices' outpatient referral rates and rates of elective admission to hospital. *British Medical Journal*, 301:273–276, 1990.

[31] D. R. Cox. Regression models and life-tables. *Journal of the Royal Statistical Society. Series B (Methodological)*, 34:187–220, 1972.

[32] D. R. Cox and D. Oakes. *Analysis of survival data*. Chapman Hall, 1st edition, 1984.

[33] J. L. Cox, J. F. Petrie, P. T. Pollak, and D. E. Johnstone. Managed delay for coronary artery bypass graft surgery: the experience at one Canadian center. *Journal of the American College of Cardiology*, 27:1365–1373, 1996.

[34] J. L. Cronenwett and R. B. Rutherford. *Decision Making in Vascular Surgery*. Saunders, 2001.

[35] C. DeCoster, K. C. Carriere, S. Peterson, R. Walld, and L. MacWilliam. Waiting times for surgical procedures. *Medical Care*, 37:JS187–JS205, 1999.

[36] E. R. DeLong, C. L. Nelson, J. B. Wong, D. B. Pryor, E. D. Peterson, K. L. Lee, D. B. Mark, R. M. Califf, and S. G. Pauker. Using observational data to estimate prognosis: an example using a coronary artery disease registry. *Statistics in Medicine*, 20:2505–2532, 2001.

[37] P. J. Diggle, K. Liang, and S. L. Zeger. *Analysis of longitudinal data*. Oxford University Press, 1st edition, 1994.

[38] B. Don, A. Lee, and M. J. Goldacre. Waiting list statistics. III. comparison of two measures of waiting times. *British Medical Journal (Clinical Research Edition)*, 295:1247–1248, 1987.

[39] J. P. Fine. Regression modeling of competing crude failure probabilities. *Biostatistics*, 2:85–97, 2001.

[40] J. P. Fine and R. J. Gray. A proportional hazards model for the subdistribution of a competing risk. *Journal of the American Statistical Association*, 94:496–509, 1999.

[41] D. M. Finkelstein, A. Muzikansky, and D. A. Schoenfeld. Comparing survival of a sample to that of a standard population. *Journal of the National Cancer Institute*, 95:1434–1439, 2003.

[42] L. D. Fisher and D. Y. Lin. Time-dependent covariates in the Cox proportional-hazards regression model. *Annual Review of Public Health*, 20:145–157, 1999.

[43] J. J. Gaynor, E. J. Feuer, C. C. Tan, D. H. Wu, C. R. Little, D. J. Straus, B. D. Clarkson, and M. F. Brennan. On the use of cause-specific failure and conditional failure probabilities - examples from clinical oncology data. *Journal of the American Statistical Association*, 88:400–409, 1993.

[44] D. H. Goldstein, E. G. VanDenKerkhof, and M. J. Rimmer. A model for real time information at the patient's side using portable computers on an acute pain service. *Canadian Journal of Anesthesia*, 49: 749–754, 2002.

[45] T. A. Gooley, W. Leisenring, J. Crowley, and B. E. Storer. Estimation of failure probabilities in the presence of competing risks: New representations of old estimators. *Statistics in Medicine*, 18: 695–706, 1999.

[46] Bob Gray. *The cmprsk Package: Subdistribution Analysis of Competing Risks*, 2004. URL http://www.r-project.org, http://biowww.dfci.harvard.edu/Ÿgray.

[47] Robert J. Gray. A class of k-sample tests for comparing the cumulative incidence of a competing risk. *The Annals of Statistics*, 16:1141–1154, 1988.

[48] R. W. Hall, editor. *Patient Flow: Reducing Delay in Healthcare Delivery*. Springer, 1st edition, 2006.

[49] D. M. Hamilton and S. Breslawski. Operating room scheduling. Factors to consider. *The Association of periOperative Registered Nurses Journal*, 59:665–680, 1994.

[50] E. L. Hannan, M. J. Racz, G. Walford, R. H. Jones, T. J. Ryan, E. Bennett, A. T. Culliford, O. W. Isom, J. P. Gold, and E. A. Rose. Long-term outcomes of coronary-artery bypass grafting versus stent implantation. *New England Journal of Medicine*, 352:2174–2183, 2005.

[51] T. R. Holford. The analysis of rates and of survivorship using log-linear models. *Biometrics*, 36: 299–305, 1980.

[52] T. R. Holford. *Multivariate Methods in Epidemiology*. Oxford University Press, 1st edition, 2002.

[53] D. W. Hosmer and S. Lemeshow. *Applied Survival Analysis: regression modeling of time to event data*, chapter Parametric Regression Models. Wiley & Son, 1st edition, 1998.

[54] D. W. Hosmer and S. Lemeshow. *Applied Survival Analysis: regression modeling of time to event data*, chapter Descriptive Methods for Survival Data, pages 27–86. Wiley & Son, 1st edition, 1998.

[55] D. W. Hosmer and S. Lemeshow. *Applied logistic regression*. John Wiley & Sons, 2nd edition, 2000.

[56] K. H. Humphries, J. M. Rankin, R. G. Carere, C. E. Buller, F. M. Kiely, and J. J. Spinelli. Co-morbidity data in outcomes research: are clinical data derived from administrative databases a reliable alternative to chart review? *Journal of Clinical Epidemiology*, 53:343–349, 2000.

[57] T. Iversen. A theory of hospital waiting lists. *Journal of Health Economics*, pages 55–71, 2000.

[58] N. W. Jackson, M. P. Doogue, and J. M. Elliott. Priority points and cardiac events while waiting for coronary bypass surgery. *Heart*, 81:367–373, 1999.

[59] J. D. Kalbfleisch and R. L. Prentice. *The statistical analysis of failure time data*. Wiley-Interscience, 2nd edition, 2002.

[60] S. J. Katz, H. F. Mizgala, and H. G. Welch. British Columbia sends patients to Seattle for coronary artery surgery. Bypassing the Queue in Canada. *Journal of the American Medical Association*, 266: 1108–1111, 1991.

[61] F. Kee, P. McDonald, J. R. Kirwan, C. C. Patterson, and A. H. Love. Urgency and priority for cardiac surgery: a clinical judgment analysis. *British Medical Journal*, 316:925–929, 1998.

[62] N. Keiding. Event history analysis and inference from observational epidemiology. *Statistics in Medicine*, 18:2353–2363, 1999.

[63] J. P. Klein. Semiparametric estimation of random effects using the Cox model based on the EM algorithm. *Biometrics*, 48:795–806, 1992.

[64] J. P. Klein and P. K. Andersen. Regression modeling of competing risks data based on pseudovalues of the cumulative incidence function. *Biometrics*, 61:223–229, 2005.

[65] J. P. Klein and M. L. Moeschberger. *Survival Analysis: Techniques for Censored and Truncated Data*, chapter Hypothesis Testing, pages 191–201. Springer, 1st edition, 1997.

[66] J. P. Klein and M. L. Moeschberger. *Survival Analysis: Techniques for Censored and Truncated Data*. Springer, 2nd edition, 2003.

[67] J. P. Klein, N. Keiding, and E. A. Copelan. Plotting summary predictions in multistate survival models: probabilities of relapse and death in remission for bone marrow transplantation patients. *Statistics in Medicine*, 12:2315–2332, 1993.

[68] E. M. Koomen, B. A. Hutten, J. C. Kelder, W. K. Redekop, J. G. Tijssen, and J. H. Kingma. Morbidity and mortality in patients waiting for coronary artery bypass surgery. *European Journal of Cardiothoracic Surgery*, 19:260–265, 2001.

[69] M. Lefkopoulou and M. Zelen. Intermediate clinical events, surrogate markers and survival. *Lifetime Data Analysis*, 1:73–85, 1995.

[70] A Levy, B Sobolev, R Hayden, M Kiely, M FitzGerald, and M Schechter. Time on wait lists for coronary bypass surgery in British Columbia, Canada, 1991 - 2000. *BMC Health Services Research*, 5:22, 2005.

[71] S. Lewis, M. L. Barer, C. Sanmartin, S. Sheps, S. E. Shortt, and P. W. McDonald. Ending waiting-list mismanagement: principles and practice [comment]. *Canadian Medical Association Journal*, 162: 1297–1300, 2000.

[72] K. Y. Liang and S. L. Zeger. Longitudinal data analysis using generalized linear models. *Biometrika*, 73:13–22, 1986.

[73] D. Y. Lin. Non-parametric inference for cumulative incidence functions in competing risks studies. *Statistics in Medicine*, 16:901–910, 1997.

[74] D. V. Lindley. *Understanding Uncertainty*. John Wiley & Sons, 1st edition, 2006.

[75] M. Lunn. Applying k-sample tests to conditional probabilities for competing risks in a clinical trial. *Biometrics*, 54:1662–1672, 1998.

[76] W. J. Mackillop, H. Fu, C. F. Quirt, P. Dixon, M. Brundage, and Y. Zhou. Waiting for radiotherapy in Ontario. *International Journal of Radiation Oncology, Biology, Physics*, 30:221–228, 1994.

[77] J. M. Magerlein and J. B. Martin. Surgical demand scheduling: a review. *Health Services Research*, 13:418–433, 1978.

[78] A. Mason. An epidemiological approach to the monitoring of hospital waiting list statistics. *Proceedings of the Royal Society of Medicine*, 69:939–942, 1976.

[79] W. McIsaac, V. Goel, and D. Naylor. Socio-economic status and visits to physicians by adults in Ontario, Canada. *Journal of Health Services Research & Policy*, 2:94–102, 1997.

[80] C. D. Morgan, K. Sykora, and C. D. Naylor. Analysis of deaths while waiting for cardiac surgery among 29,293 consecutive patients in Ontario, Canada. *Heart*, 79:345–349, 1998.

[81] C. D. Naylor. A different view of queues in Ontario. *Health Affairs*, 10:110–128, 1991.

[82] C. D. Naylor, R. S. Baigrie, B. S. Goldman, and A. Basinski. Assessment of priority for coronary revascularisation procedures. *Lancet*, 335:1070–1073, 1990.

[83] C. D. Naylor, C. M. Levinton, and R. S. Baigrie. Adapting to waiting lists for coronary revascularization. Do Canadian specialists agree on which patients come first? *Chest*, 101:715–722, 1992.

[84] C. D. Naylor, K. Sykora, S. B. Jaglal, and S. Jefferson. Waiting for coronary artery bypass surgery: population-based study of 8517 consecutive patients in Ontario, Canada. the steering committee of the adult cardiac care network of Ontario [see comments]. *Lancet*, 346:1605–1609, 1995.

[85] J. A. Nelder and R. W. M. Wedderburn. Generalized linear models. *Journal of the Royal Statistical Society A*, 135:370–384, 1972.

[86] T. W. Noseworthy, J. J. McGurran, and D. C. Hadorn. Waiting for scheduled services in Canada: development of priority-setting scoring systems. *Journal of Evaluation in Clinical Practice*, 9:23–31, 2003.

[87] N. J. O'Connor, J. R. Morton, J. D. Birkmeyer, E. M. Olmstead, and G. T. O'Connor. Effect of coronary artery diameter in patients undergoing coronary bypass surgery. Northern New England Cardiovascular Disease Study Group. *Circulation*, 93:652–655, 1996.

[88] J. P. Pell, A. C. Pell, J. Norrie, I. Ford, and S. M. Cobbe. Effect of socioeconomic deprivation on waiting time for cardiac surgery: retrospective cohort study. *British Medical Journal*, 320:15–18, 2000.

[89] M. S. Pepe. Inference for events with dependent risks in multiple end-point studies. *Journal of the American Statistical Association*, 86:770–778, 1991.

[90] M. S. Pepe and M. Mori. Kaplan-Meier, marginal or conditional-probability curves in summarizing competing risks failure time data. *Statistics in Medicine*, 12:737–751, 1993.

[91] M. Pintilie. *Competing Risks: A Practical Perspective*. John Wiley & Sons, 1st edition, 2006.

[92] J. Plomp, W. K. Redekop, F. W. Dekker, T. R. van Geldorp, M. M. Haalebos, G. Jambroes, J. H. Kingma, F. Zijlstra, and J. G. Tijssen. Death on the waiting list for cardiac surgery in the Netherlands in 1994 and 1995. *Heart*, 81:593–597, 1999.

[93] R. L. Prentice and L. A. Gloeckler. Regression analysis of grouped survival data with application to breast cancer data. *Biometrics*, 34:57–67, 1978.

[94] A. A. Ray, K. J. Buth, J. A. Sullivan, D. E. Johnstone, and G. M. Hirsch. Waiting for cardiac surgery: results of a risk-stratified queuing process. *Circulation*, 104:I92–I98, 2001.

[95] H. Rexius, G. Brandrup-Wognsen, A. Oden, and A. Jeppsson. Mortality on the waiting list for coronary artery bypass grafting: incidence and risk factors. *Annals of Thoracic Surgery*, 77:769–774, 2004.

[96] C. S. Rihal, D. L. Raco, B. J. Gersh, and S. Yusuf. Indications for coronary artery bypass surgery and percutaneous coronary intervention in chronic stable angina: review of the evidence and methodological considerations. *Circulation*, 108:2439–2445, 2003.

[97] P. S. Romano, L. L. Roos, and J. G. Jollis. Adapting a clinical comorbidity index for use with ICD-9-CM administrative data: differing perspectives. *Journal of Clinical Epidemiology*, 46:1075–1079, 1993.

[98] N. P. Roos and C. A. Mustard. Variation in health and health care use by socioeconomic status in Winnipeg, Canada: does the system work well? Yes and no. *The Milbank Quarterly*, 75:89–111, 1997.

[99] C. Sanmartin, S. E. Shortt, M. L. Barer, S. Sheps, S. Lewis, and P. W. McDonald. Waiting for medical services in Canada: lots of heat, but little light. *Canadian Medical Association Journal*, 162:1305–1310, 2000.

[100] T. Scheike and T. K Jensen. A discrete survival model with random effects: an application to time to pregnancy. *Biometrics*, 53:318–329, 1997.

[101] M. E. Seddon, J. K. French, D. J. Amos, K. Ramanathan, S. C. McLaughlin, and H. D. White. Waiting times and prioritization for coronary artery bypass surgery in New Zealand. *Heart*, 81:586–592, 1999.

[102] J. D. Singer and J. B. Willett. *Applied Longitudinal Data Analysis: modeling change and event occurrence*, chapter The person-level data set, pages 19–23. Oxford University Press, 2003.

[103] B. Sobolev, P. Brown, and D. Zelt. Variation in time spent on the waiting list for elective vascular surgery: a case study. *Clinical and Investigative Medicine*, 23:227–238, 2000.

[104] B. Sobolev, P. Brown, D. Zelt, and S. Shortt. Bias inherent in retrospective waiting-time studies: experience from a vascular surgery waiting list. *Canadian Medical Association Journal*, 162:1821–1822, 2000.

[105] B. Sobolev, P. Brown, and D. Zelt. Potential for bias in waiting-time studies: events between enrolment and admission. *Journal of Epidemiology and Community Health*, 55:891–894, 2001.

[106] B. Sobolev, P. Brown, and D. Zelt. Modeling and analysis of multistate access to elective surgery. *Health Care Management Science*, 4:125–132, 2001.

[107] B. Sobolev, P. Brown, D. Zelt, and S. Shortt. Access to elective vascular surgery within the recommended time according to emergency referrals. *Clinical and Investigative Medicine*, 24:236–241, 2001.

[108] B. Sobolev, D. Mercer, P. Brown, J. M. FitzGerald, D. Jalink, and R. Shaw. Risk of emergency admission while awaiting elective cholecystectomy. *Canadian Medical Association Journal*, 169:662–665, 2003.

[109] B. Sobolev, P. Brown, D. Zelt, and L. Kuramoto. Waiting time in relation to wait-list size at registration: statistical Analysis of a waiting-list registry. *Clinical and Investigative Medicine*, 27:298–305, 2004.

[110] B. Sobolev, A. Levy, and L. Kuramoto. Summarizing the probability of wait-list events. *Journal of Evaluation in Clinical Practice*, 11:606–608, 2005.

[111] B. Sobolev, L. Kuramoto, A. Levy, and R. Hayden. Cumulative incidence for wait-list death in relation to length of queue for coronary-artery bypass grafting: a cohort study. *Journal of Cardiothoracic Surgery*, 1:22, 2006.

[112] B. Sobolev, A. Levy, R. Hayden, and L. Kuramoto. Does wait-list size at registration influence time to surgery? Analysis of a population-based cardiac surgery registry. *Health Services Research*, 41:23–39, 2006.

[113] B. Sobolev, A. Levy, L. Kuramoto, and R. Hayden. Unplanned emergency admission in relation to length of wait lists at registration. *Clinical and Investigative Medicine*, 29:193–200, 2006.

[114] B. G. Sobolev, M. D. Brown, D. Zelt, and J. M. FitzGerald. Priority waiting lists: Is there a clinically ordered queue? *Journal of Evaluation in Clinical Practice*, 11:408–410, 2005.

[115] B. G. Sobolev, A. R. Levy, L. Kuramoto, and R. Hayden. Chances of late surgery in relation to length of wait lists. *BMC Health Services Research*, 5:63, 2005.

[116] B. G. Sobolev, A. R. Levy, L. Kuramoto, R. Hayden, J. M. Brophy, and J. M. FitzGerald. The risk of death associated with delayed coronary artery bypass surgery. *BMC Health Services Research*, 6:85, 2006.

[117] B. G Sobolev, A. R. Levy, L. Kuramoto, R. Hayden, and J. M. FitzGerald. Do longer delays for coronary bypass surgery contribute to pre-operative mortality in less urgent patients? *Medical Care*, 44:680–686, 2006.

[118] K. Sykora, P. M. Slaughter, W. Young, D Garlin, and C. D. Naylor. *Cardiovascular Health and Services in Ontario: An ICES Atlas*, chapter Waiting lists for cardiac surgery, pages 239–254. Institute for Clinical Evaluative Sciences, 1999.

[119] S. J. Thomas, M. V. Williams, N. G. Burnet, and C. R. Baker. How much surplus capacity is required to maintain low waiting times? *Clinical Oncology (Royal College of Radiologists (Great Britain))*, 13:24–28, 2001.

[120] T. Volk, L. Hahn, R. Hayden, J. Abel, M. L. Puterman, and G. F. Tyers. Reliability audit of a regional cardiac surgery registry. *Journal of Thoracic and Cardiovascular Surgery*, 114:903–910, 1997.

[121] C. R. Weinberg, D. D. Baird, and A. S. Rowland. Pitfalls inherent in retrospective time-to-event studies: the example of time to pregnancy. *Statistics in Medicine*, 12:867–879, 1993.

[122] S. Yusuf, D. Zucker, P. Peduzzi, L. D. Fisher, T. Takaro, J. W. Kennedy, K. Davis, T. Killip, E. Passamani, and R. Norris. Effect of coronary artery bypass graft surgery on survival: overview of 10-year results from randomised trials by the coronary artery bypass graft surgery trialists collaboration. *Lancet*, 344:563–570, 1994.

Index

CPSIA information can be obtained at www.ICGtesting.com
Printed in the USA
LVOW130950091011

249706LV00002B/3/A

9 780387 764214